MEMORY NOTEBOOK OF NURSING
Volume 1, 5th Edition

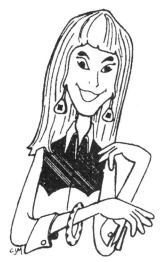

JoAnn Zerwekh, EdD, MSN, RN
President/CEO
Nursing Education Consultants
Chandler, AZ

Nursing Faculty
University of Phoenix
Phoenix, AZ

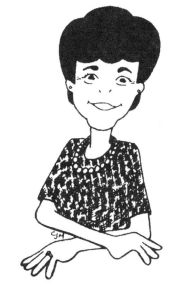

Jo Carol Claborn, MS, RN

Nursing Education Consultants

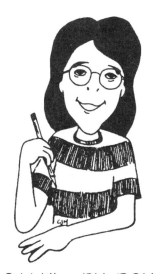

CJ Miller, RN, BSN

Nurse Illustrator
Cedar Rapids, IA

Artist: C.J. Miller, RN, BSN
Cedar Rapids, IA

Production Manager: Mike Cull
Gingerbread Press, Waxahachie, TX
Desktop Publishing: Lindy Nobles, Prosper, TX

◆

◆

Printed in the United States of America

Nursing Education Consultants
P O Box 12200
Chandler, AZ 85248
www.NursingEd.com

ISBN 9781892155184
LOC #: 2011939043

◆

Any procedure or practice described in this book should be applied by the health-care practitioner und appropriate supervision in accordance with professional standards of care used with regard to the uniqu circumstances that apply in each practice situation. Care has been taken to confirm the accuracy of informatic presented and to describe generally accepted practices. However, the authors, editors, and publisher cannc accept any responsibility for errors or omissions or for consequences from application of the information in th book and make no warranty, express or implied, with respect to the contents of this book.

This book is written to be used as a study aid and review book for nursing. It is not intended for use as a primar resource for procedures, treatments, medications or to serve as a complete textbook for nursing care.

Copies of this book may be obtained directly from your local textbook store, or directly from Nursing Educatic Consultants (http:www.nursinged.com).

Last Digit Is the Print Number: 6 5 4 3 2

CONTRIBUTORS

Joanna Barnes, MSN, RN
ADN Program Director
Grayson County College
Denison, TX

Deanne A. Blach, MSN, RN
Nurse Educator
President, DB Productions
Green Forest, AR

Tim Bristol, PhD, RN, CNE
NurseTim, Inc.
Executive Director
Waconia, MN

Sharon Decker, PhD, RN, ACNS-BC, ANEF
Professor and Director of Clinical Simulations
Covenant Health System Endowed Chair in
Simulation and Nursing Education
Texas Tech University Health Science Center
Lubbock, TX

Barbara Devitt, MSN, RN
Nursing Faculty
Louise Herrington School of Nursing
Baylor University
Dallas, TX

Debra L. Fontenot, DNP, RN, CPNP, CNE
Instructor
Alvin Community College
Alvin, TX

Shirley Greenway, MSN, RN
Instructor
Grayson County College
Denison, TX

Lt. Col. (Ret.) Michael W. Hutton, MSN, RN
Nursing Faculty
Blinn College
Bryan, TX

Catherine Rosser, EdD, RN, CAN-BC,
Undergraduate Program Director
Louise Herrington School of Nursing
Baylor University
Dallas, TX

Virginia "Ginny" Wangerin, RN, MSN, PhDc
Nurse Consultant, Educator
Administrator Emeritus,
Des Moines Area Community College
President, Iowa Nurses Association, 2007-2011

Mary Ann Yantis, BS, MS, PhD, RN
Faculty
Nursing Education Consultants, Inc.
Chandler, AZ

2012 Nursing Education
nsultants, Inc.

Memory Notebook of Nursing, Vol. 1 - 5th ed.
NursingEd.com

iii

ACKNOWLEDGMENTS

From the authors: We want to express our appreciation to the students and faculty who have responded so positively to the *Memory Notebook of Nursing, Vol 1*. Through your support and contributions, this 5th edition was possible.

We wish to thank Robert Claborn and John Masog (our husbands) for their tolerance and sense of humor as we continued to work on revisions of another book! Also, we want to thank our 'adult children' Ashley Garneau and Tyler Zerwekh, Jaelyn Conway, Mike Brown, and Kimberley Aultman for their unconditional support and inspiration as we continue our journey in publishing.

From the illustrator: My work is dedicated to Nathan and Kim, the two best kids in the world and to my grandson Cohen. Without your love and support, I couldn't do what I do.

Our sincere appreciation to:

Lindy Nobles, our graphics production manager, who's exceptional technological skills contributed to the major revision of this project;

Mike Cull and all the support staff at CuLeGo for their persistence and patience in working with us;

Elaine Nokes for keeping our office running smoothly while we are busy revising our books;

Dave Meier from the Center for Accelerated Learning at Lake Geneva, WI for introducing us to these ideas to help students learn.

iv

Memory Notebook of Nursing, Vol. 1 - 5th ed.
NursingEd.com

PREFACE

Memory Notebook of Nursing, Volume 1 was the first of the series of Memory Notebooks of Nursing. We are so pleased that you have enjoyed the images and mnemonics over the years and we are excited to bring you this 5th edition. This one, as the last, continues to utilize the unique visual approach to learning. This edition will continue to assist you in studying, reviewing, and presenting information. It is a great tool for the nursing student who is struggling through the enormous amount of material in nursing school, as well as for the new graduate who is preparing for the National Council Licensure Exam (NCLEX). Nursing Education Consultants has continued to utilize the principles of accelerated learning and humorous visual images to provide and appealing and engaging approach to remember important information. This learning strategy is made possible by the illustrations of C.J. Miller, who is also a nurse.

First, a little information about accelerated learning and how you can enhance your learning by utilizing both the left (analytical, linear, logical, rote memory) side of your brain and the right (visual, images, musical, imaginative) side of your brain. Several techniques are used to encourage the whole-brain to think and learn concepts. These techniques are memory tools, mindmapping, and mnemonics. Memory tools are aids to assist you to draw associations from other ideas with the use of visual images to help cement the learning. Mindmapping (or concept mapping) is a tool to help people take notes more effectively. Mindmapping is in sharp contrast to the traditional method of taking notes in an outline format. Instead, a thought or concept is written in the center of the page, images and color are added to information as ideas begin to flow out from the center focus. Another technique is the use of mnemonics. Mnemonics are most often words, phrases, or sentences that help you remember information. Throughout this book, you will find ideas that we have found useful in teaching students how to remember information. As you read over each illustration, get involved with the process and write down your own ideas on the drawings. Think about this, color activates the brain and music increases right brain activity. Time to get out the crayolas or colored pencils and color the pictures. As you are coloring or writing, turn on some music, don't be afraid to experiment – find out what type of music works best for you.

If you really like the *Memory Notebook of Nursing, Vol 1, 5th edition*, then check out other Memory Notebooks of Nursing. *Memory Notebook of Nursing, Vol 2, 4th edition* has more great images and mnemonics, and *Memory Notebook of Nursing: Pharmacology & Diagnostics, 2nd edition* provides a great study guide for pharmacology and diagnostic tests. Same great concepts — different images and mnemonics in all three books. On the inside of the back cover, you will find more information about these helpful study aids.

The authors of this book also have NCLEX review books for both PNs and RNs. These texts can be ordered from Nursing Education Consultants, Inc. website — http://www.nursinged.com. The comments from Nursing Education Consultants' Review course participants, our students, and other nursing faculty have helped to shape the development of these review texts.

JoAnn Zerwekh

Jo Carol Claborn

2012 Nursing Education
Consultants, Inc.

Memory Notebook of Nursing, Vol. 1 - 5th ed.
NursingEd.com

V

vi

Memory Notebook of Nursing, Vol. 1 - 5th ed.
NursingEd.com

© 2012 Nursing Educatio
Consultants, In

TABLE OF CONTENTS

2012 Nursing Education
nsultants, Inc.

Memory Notebook of Nursing, Vol. 1 - 5th ed.
NursingEd.com

vii

ABNORMAL CELL GROWTH

PSYCHOSOCIAL NURSING CONCEPTS

SENSORY

ENDOCRINE

HEMATOLOGY

RESPIRATORY

Memory Notebook of Nursing, Vol. 1 - 5th ed.
NursingEd.com

© 2012 Nursing Education
Consultants, Inc

2012 Nursing Education
nsultants, Inc.

Memory Notebook of Nursing, Vol. 1 - 5th ed.
NursingEd.com

ix

Memory Notebook of Nursing, Vol. 1 - 5th ed.
NursingEd.com

© 2012 Nursing Educati
Consultants, Ir

COMPUTER ADAPTIVE TESTING

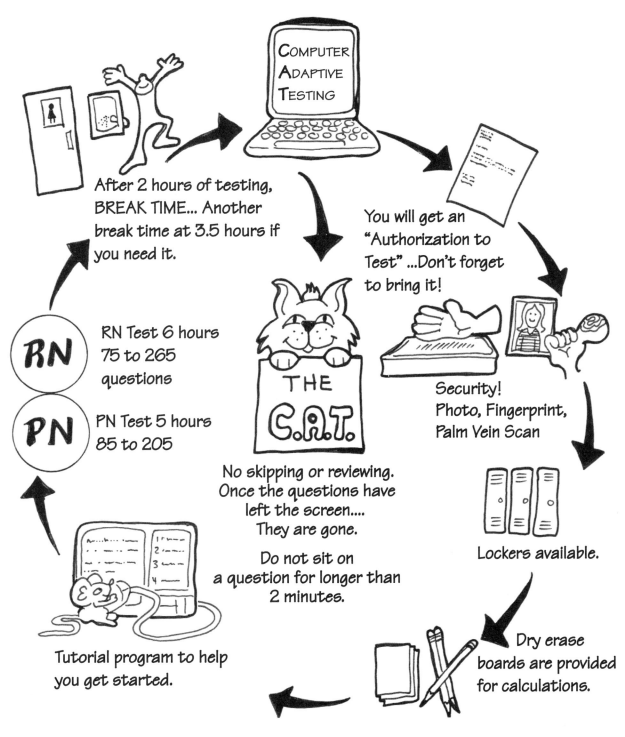

After 2 hours of testing, BREAK TIME... Another break time at 3.5 hours if you need it.

RN Test 6 hours 75 to 265 questions

PN Test 5 hours 85 to 205

You will get an "Authorization to Test" ...Don't forget to bring it!

Security! Photo, Fingerprint, Palm Vein Scan

THE C.A.T.

No skipping or reviewing. Once the questions have left the screen.... They are gone.

Do not sit on a question for longer than 2 minutes.

Lockers available.

Dry erase boards are provided for calculations.

Tutorial program to help you get started.

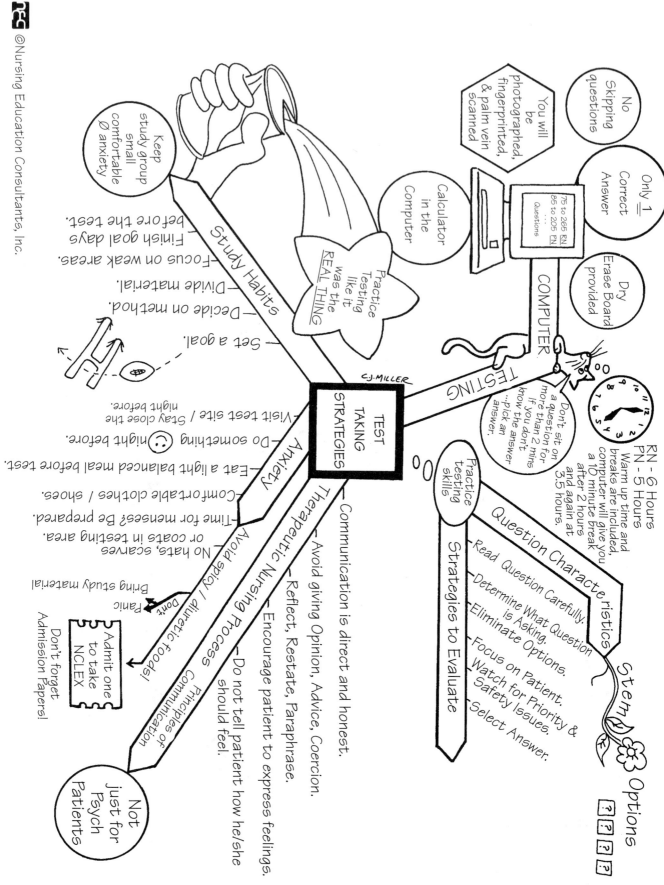

TEST TAKING STRATEGIES

Study Habits
- Set a goal.
- Decide on method.
- Divide material.
- Focus on weak areas.
- Finish goal days before the test.

Keep study group small comfortable Ø anxiety

Practice Testing like it was the REAL THING

COMPUTER TESTING
You will be photographed, fingerprinted, & palm vein scanned

75 to 265 RN / 85 to 205 PN Questions

Calculator in the Computer

No Skipping questions

Only 1 Correct Answer

Dry Erase Board provided

Don't sit on a question for more than 2 mins. If you don't know the answer...pick an answer.

RN - 6 Hours
PN - 5 Hours
Warm up time and breaks are included, computer will give you a 10 minute break after 2 hours and again at 3.5 hours.

Practice testing skills

Question Characteristics
Strategies to Evaluate
- Read Question Carefully.
- Determine What Question is Asking.
- Eliminate Options.
- Focus on Patient.
- Watch for Priority & Safety Issues.
- Select Answer.

Stem
Options
[?] [?] [?]
[?]

Anxiety
- Visit test site / Stay close the night before.
- Do something ☺ night before.
- Eat a light balanced meal before test.
- Comfortable clothes / shoes.
- Time for menses? Be prepared.
- No hats, scarves or coats in testing area.

Panic
Don't Bring study material

Admit one to take NCLEX

Don't forget Admission Papers!

Avoid spicy / diuretic foods!

Therapeutic Nursing Process
Principles of Communication
- Communication is direct and honest.
- Avoid giving Opinion, Advice, Coercion.
- Reflect, Restate, Paraphrase.
- Encourage patient to express feelings.
- Do not tell patient how he/she should feel.

Not just for Psych Patients

CJ. MILLER

MASLOW'S HIERARCHY OF BASIC HUMAN NEEDS

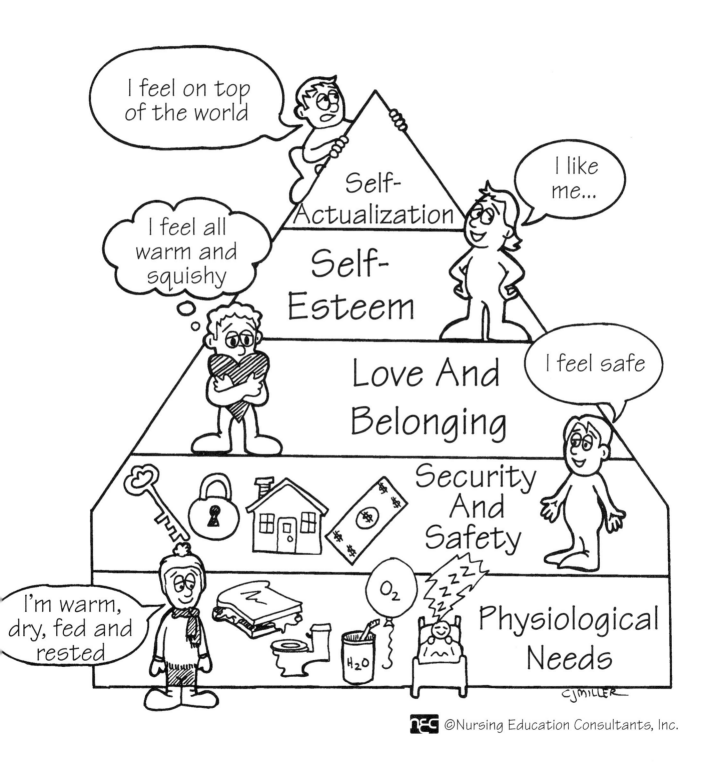

STEPS IN THE NURSING PROCESS

A Delicious PIE:

Assessment
Diagnosis
Planning
Implementation
Evaluation

An Apple PIE:

Assessment
Analysis
Planning
Implementation
Evaluation

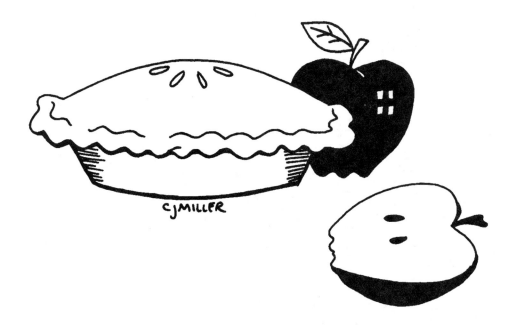

CJMILLER

Concepts of Nursing Practice
NursingEd.com

© 2012 Nursing Educat...
Consultants,

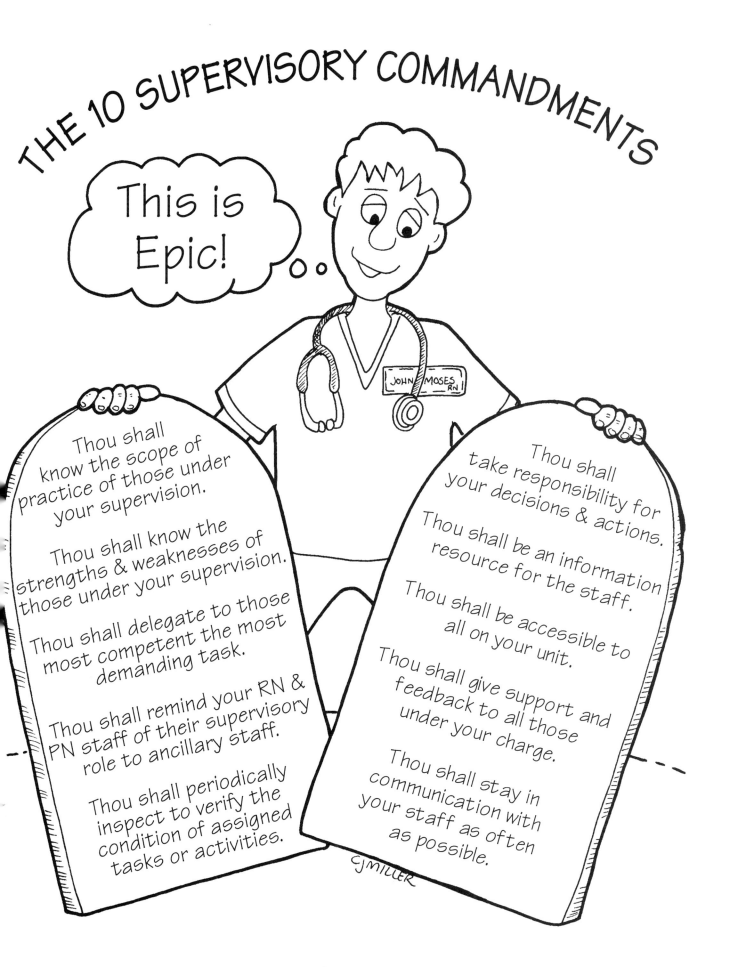

CHARTING BODY FLUIDS
"Coach"

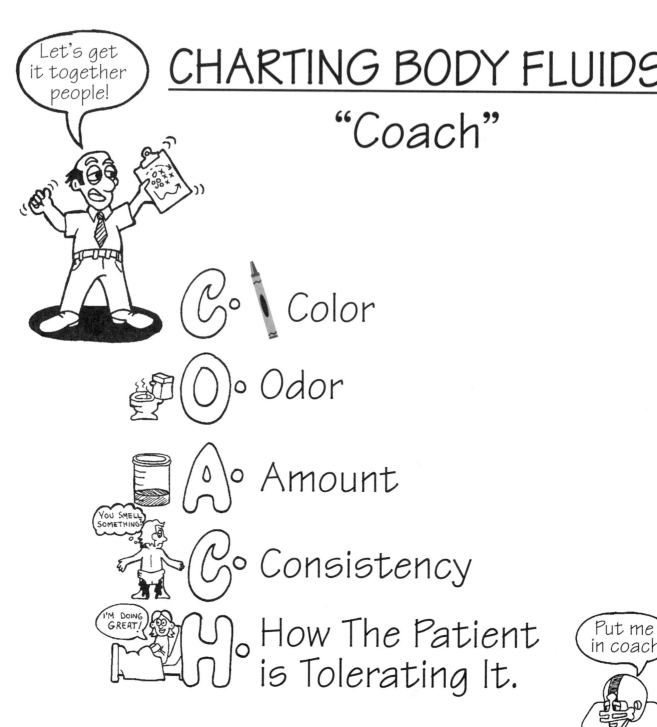

C° Color

O° Odor

A° Amount

C° Consistency

H° How The Patient is Tolerating It.

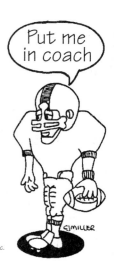

Concepts of Nursing Practice
NursingEd.com

CARE OF THE CHRONICALLY ILL CHILD

Most Common Chronic Childhood Conditions –
1. Respiratory (Asthma)
2. Speech and Sensory Impairments
3. Mental and Nervous System Disorders

Decline in mortality rate increases in number of children with special health care needs.

Focus on child's developmental age not chronological age.

Promote, Maintain, or Restore Health.

Maximize independence while minimizing effects of chronic condition.

Family Centered Care:
Assess family response to illness

Involve family in care

Assist family to promote maximum growth and development

CJ MILLER

Hospitalization –
- Determine how child is cared for at home & maintain routines
- Respect family's expertise in care of child
- Be attentive to parents' or caregiver's input
- Care conferences for planning & sharing mutual concerns
- Encourage independence and self-care

MEDICAL ASEPSIS

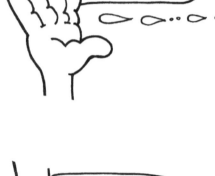

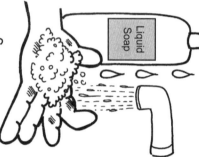

Hand Hygiene is number ☆1

- Reduces number of pathogens

- Referred to as "Clean technique"

- Used in administration of:
  Medications
  Enemas
  Tube feedings
  Daily hygiene

SURGICAL ASEPSIS

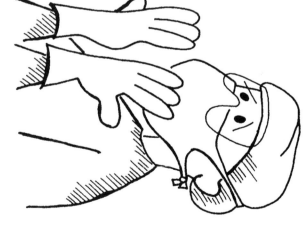

- Eliminates all pathogens

- Referred to as "Sterile technique"

- Used in:
  Dressing changes
  Catheterizations
  Surgical Procedures

C.J. MILLER

 ©Nursing Education Consultants, Inc.

PRE OP CHECKLIST
DAY OF SURGERY

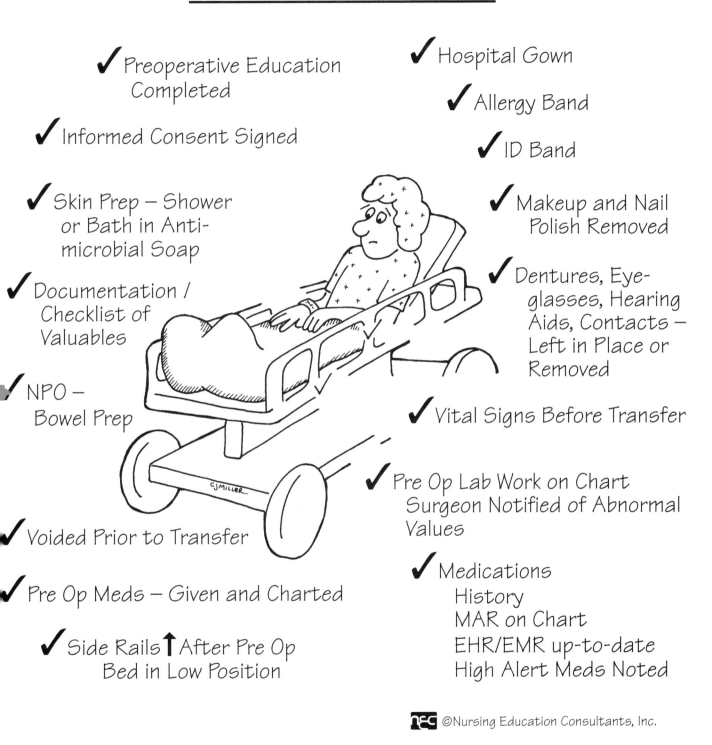

✔ Preoperative Education Completed

✔ Informed Consent Signed

✔ Skin Prep – Shower or Bath in Anti-microbial Soap

✔ Documentation / Checklist of Valuables

✔ NPO – Bowel Prep

✔ Voided Prior to Transfer

✔ Pre Op Meds – Given and Charted

✔ Side Rails ↑ After Pre Op Bed in Low Position

✔ Hospital Gown

✔ Allergy Band

✔ ID Band

✔ Makeup and Nail Polish Removed

✔ Dentures, Eye-glasses, Hearing Aids, Contacts – Left in Place or Removed

✔ Vital Signs Before Transfer

✔ Pre Op Lab Work on Chart Surgeon Notified of Abnormal Values

✔ Medications
    History
    MAR on Chart
    EHR/EMR up-to-date
    High Alert Meds Noted

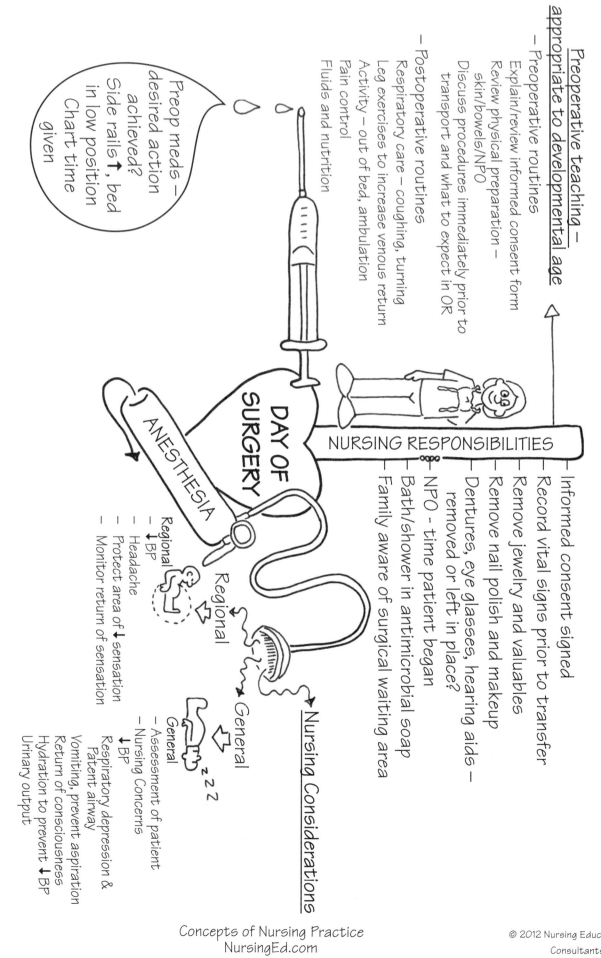

Preoperative teaching – appropriate to developmental age

– Preoperative routines
  Explain/review informed consent form
  Review physical preparation – skin/bowels/NPO
  Discuss procedures immediately prior to transport and what to expect in OR

– Postoperative routines
  Respiratory care – coughing, turning
  Leg exercises to increase venous return
  Activity – out of bed, ambulation
  Pain control
  Fluids and nutrition

Preop meds – desired action achieved?
Side rails ↑, bed in low position
Chart time given

DAY OF SURGERY

ANESTHESIA

Regional
– ↓ BP
– Headache
– Protect area of ↓ sensation
– Monitor return of sensation

Regional

Regional

General
– Assessment of patient
– Nursing Concerns
  ↓ BP
  Respiratory depression & patent airway
  Vomiting, prevent aspiration
  Return of consciousness
  Hydration to prevent ↓ BP
  Urinary output

General

General

NURSING RESPONSIBILITIES

– Informed consent signed
– Record vital signs prior to transfer
– Remove jewelry and valuables
– Remove nail polish and makeup
– Dentures, eye glasses, hearing aids – removed or left in place?
– NPO - time patient began
– Bath/shower in antimicrobial soap
– Family aware of surgical waiting area

Nursing Considerations

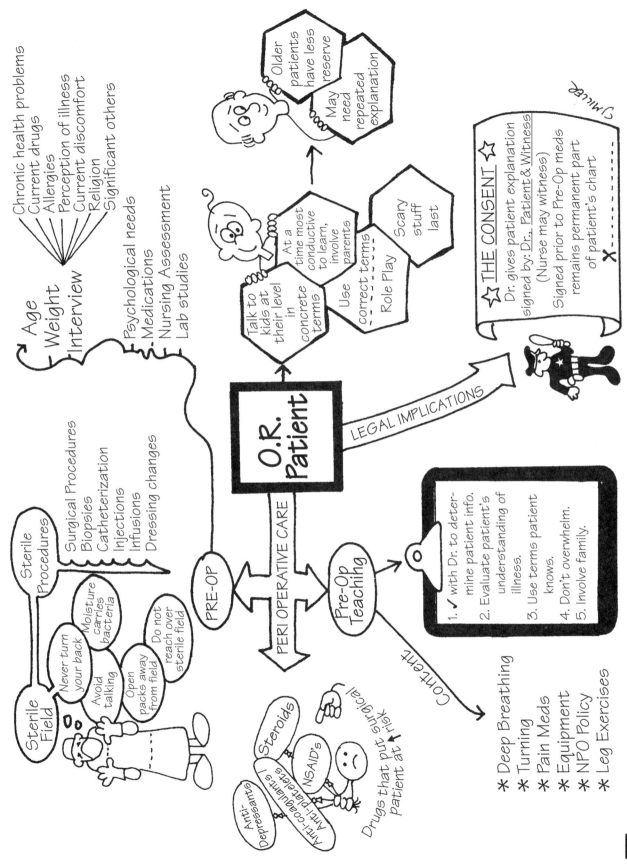

O.R. Patient

PERI OPERATIVE CARE

Interview
Age
Weight
Chronic health problems
Current drugs
Allergies
Perception of illness
Current discomfort
Religion
Significant others

Psychological needs
Medications
Nursing Assessment
Lab studies

Older patients have less reserve
May need repeated explanation

Talk to kids at their level in concrete terms
At a time most conductive to learn, involve parents
Use correct terms
Role Play
Scary stuff last

☆ THE CONSENT ☆
Dr. gives patient explanation
signed by: Dr., Patient & Witness
(Nurse may witness)
Signed prior to Pre-Op meds
remains permanent part
of patient's chart
CJMILLER

LEGAL IMPLICATIONS

PRE-OP

Sterile Procedures
Surgical Procedures
Biopsies
Catheterization
Injections
Infusions
Dressing changes

Sterile Field
Never turn your back
Moisture carries bacteria
Avoid talking
Open packs away from field
Do not reach over sterile field

Drugs that put surgical Patient at risk
Steroids
NSAID's
Anti-coagulants
Anti-platelets
Anti-Depressants

Pre-Op Teaching
1. ✓ with Dr. to determine patient info.
2. Evaluate patient's understanding of illness.
3. Use terms patient knows.
4. Don't overwhelm.
5. Involve family.

Content
* Deep Breathing
* Turning
* Pain Meds
* Equipment
* NPO Policy
* Leg Exercises

©Nursing Education Consultants, Inc.

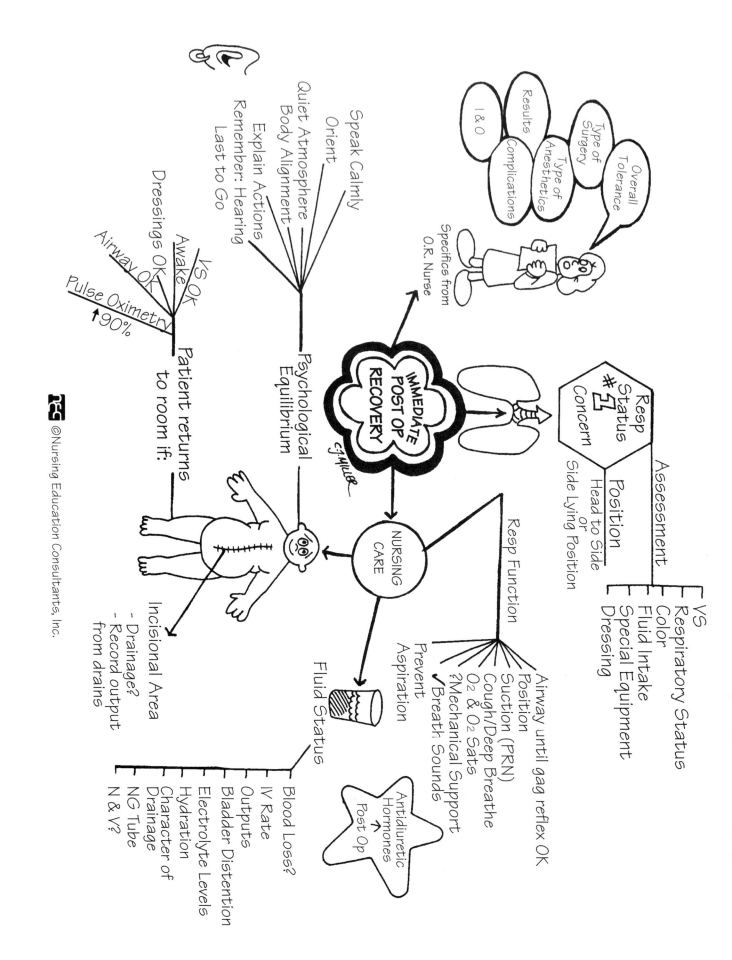

IMMEDIATE POST OP RECOVERY
CJ Miller

Psychological Equilibrium
- Speak Calmly
- Quiet Atmosphere
- Orient
- Body Alignment
- Explain Actions
- Remember: Hearing Last to Go

Patient returns to room if:
- Awake
- VS Ok
- Airway OK
- Dressings OK
- Pulse Oximetry ↑ 90%

Specifics from O.R. Nurse
- I & O
- Results
- Complications
- Type of Anesthetics
- Type of Surgery
- Overall Tolerance

Resp Status #1 Concern
- Position Head to Side or Side Lying Position
- Assessment
  - VS
  - Respiratory Status
  - Color
  - Fluid Intake
  - Special Equipment
  - Dressing

NURSING CARE

Resp Function
- Prevent Aspiration
- Airway until gag reflex OK
- Position
- Suction (PRN)
- Cough/Deep Breathe
- O₂ & O₂ Sats
- ?Mechanical Support
- ✓Breath Sounds

Antidiuretic Hormones → Post Op

Incisional Area
- Drainage?
- Record output from drains

Fluid Status
- Blood Loss?
- IV Rate
- Outputs
- Bladder Distention
- Electrolyte Levels
- Hydration
- Character of Drainage
- NG Tube
- N & V?

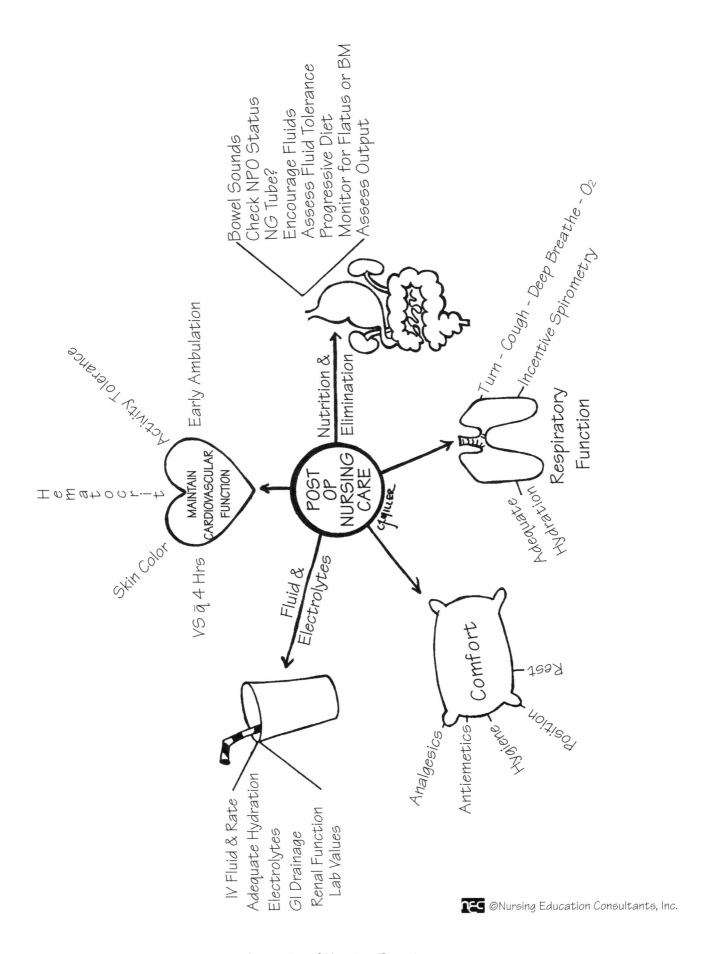

POST OP NURSING CARE

Nutrition & Elimination
- Bowel Sounds
- Check NPO Status
- NG Tube?
- Encourage Fluids
- Assess Fluid Tolerance
- Progressive Diet
- Monitor for Flatus or BM
- Assess Output

Maintain Cardiovascular Function
- Activity Tolerance
- Early Ambulation
- Hematocrit
- Skin Color
- VS q̄ 4 Hrs

Respiratory Function
- Turn - Cough - Deep Breathe - O$_2$
- Incentive Spirometry
- Adequate Hydration

Comfort
- Rest
- Position
- Hygiene
- Antiemetics
- Analgesics

Fluid & Electrolytes
- IV Fluid & Rate
- Adequate Hydration
- Electrolytes
- GI Drainage
- Renal Function Lab Values

©Nursing Education Consultants, Inc.

POST OP COMPLICATIONS

URINARY RETENTION
- Should Void Within 6-8 Hrs Post Op
- Palpable Bladder
- Frequent, Small Amount Voiding
- Pain Suprapubic Area

PNEUMONIA
- Rapid Shallow Respirations
- Fever
- Wet Breath Sounds
- Asymmetrical Chest Movement
- Productive Cough
- Hypoxia
- Tachycardia
- Leukocytosis

ATELECTASIS
- Dyspnea
- ↓O₂ Sats & ↓PaO₂
- ↓Breath Sounds
- Asymmetrical Chest Movement
- ↑Tachycardia
- ↑Restlessness

URINARY

RESPIRATORY

PULMONARY EMBOLISM
- Chest Pain
- Dyspnea
- ↑Resp Rate
- Tachycardia
- ↑Anxiety
- Diaphoresis
- ↓Orientation
- ↓BP
- Blood Gas Changes

CIRCULATORY

HYPOVOLEMIC SHOCK
- ↓Urine
- ↓BP
- Weak Pulse
- Cool Clammy
- Restless
- ↑Bleeding
- ↑Thirst

PARALYTIC ILEUS
- ↓Bowel Sounds
- No Stool or Flatus
- Nausea
- Vomiting
- Abd Distention
- Abd Tenderness

GASTRIC DILATION
- Nausea & Vomiting
- Abd Distention

EVISCERATION
- Evidence of Bowel Through Incision
- ↑Pain

DEHISCENCE
- Separation of Incision

INFECTION
- Redness
- Purulent Drainage
- Fever
- Tachycardia
- Leukocytosis

Concepts of Nursing Practice
NursingEd.com

© 2012 Nursing Educati
Consultants, In

DEHISCENCE / EVISCERATION

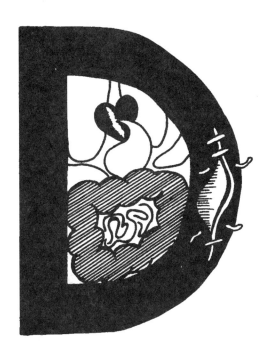

Dehiscence

Separation or splitting open of layers of a surgical wound

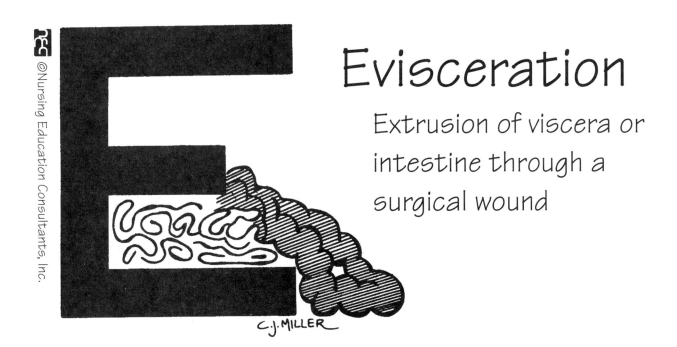

Evisceration

Extrusion of viscera or intestine through a surgical wound

C.J. MILLER

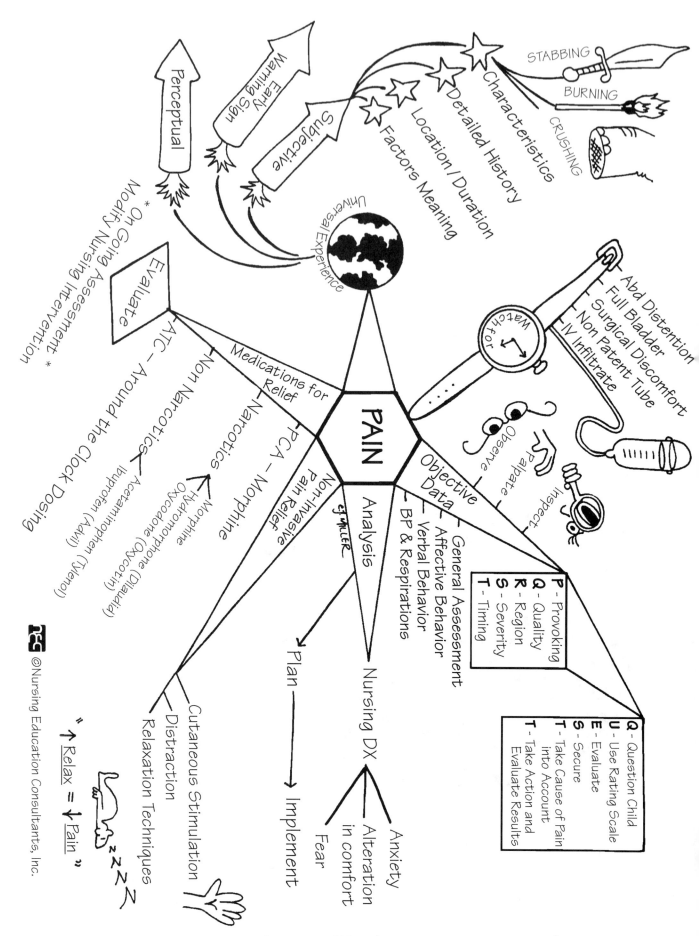

PAIN

STABBING
BURNING
CRUSHING

Characteristics
Detailed History
Location / Duration
Factors Meaning

Subjective
Early Warning Sign
Perceptual

Universal Experience

* Modify Nursing Intervention *
* On Going Assessment *
Evaluate

Medications for Relief

Non Narcotics — ATC – Around the Clock Dosing
Acetaminophen (Tylenol)
Ibuprofen (Advil)

Narcotics
Oxycodone (Oxycontin)
Hydromorphone (Dilaudid)
Morphine
PCA – Morphine

Non-Invasive Pain Relief

Analysis

Objective Data

Abd Distention
Full Bladder
Surgical Discomfort
Non Patent Tube
IV Infiltrate

Watch for
Observe
Palpate
Inspect

BP & Respirations
Verbal Behavior
Affective Behavior
General Assessment

P - Provoking
Q - Quality
R - Region
S - Severity
T - Timing

Q - Question Child
U - Use Rating Scale
E - Evaluate
S - Secure
T - Take Cause of Pain into Account
T - Take Action and Evaluate Results

Relaxation Techniques
Distraction
Cutaneous Stimulation

Plan → Implement

Nursing DX
Anxiety
Alteration in comfort
Fear

" ↑ Relax = ↓ Pain "

CJ MILLER

Concepts of Nursing Practice
NursingEd.com

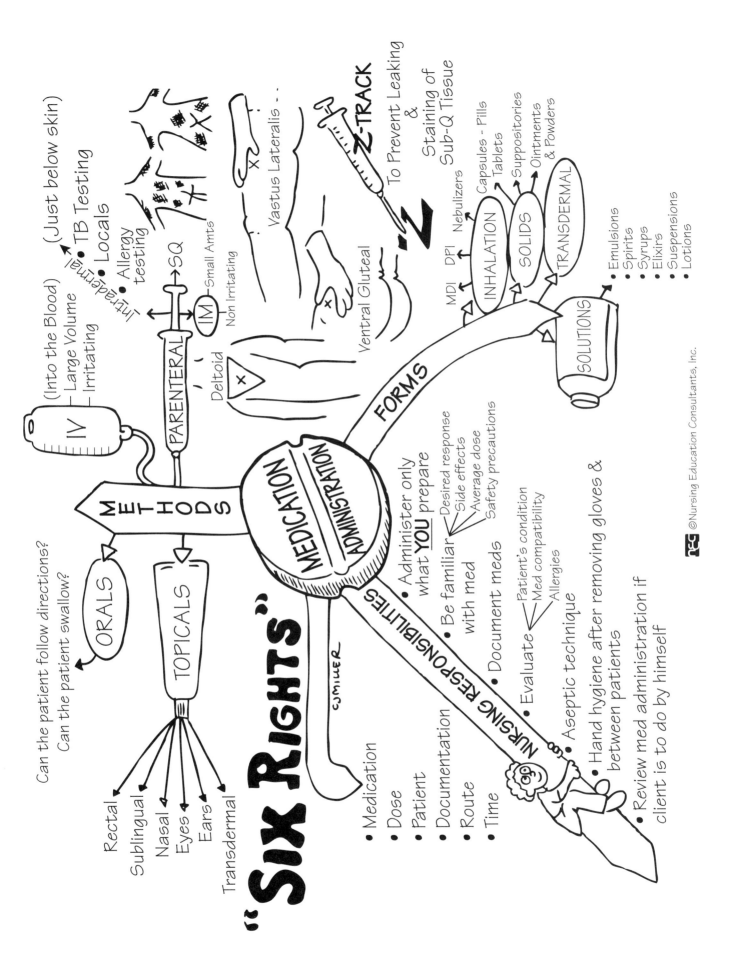

"Six Rights"

MEDICATION ADMINISTRATION

- Medication
- Dose
- Patient
- Documentation
- Route
- Time

METHODS

IV — (Into the Blood)
— Large Volume
— Irritating

PARENTERAL → SQ (Just below skin)
Intradermal
• TB Testing
• Locals
• Allergy testing

IM — Small Amts
— Non Irritating

Deltoid
Vastus Lateralis
Ventral Gluteal

Z-TRACK
To Prevent Leaking & Staining of Sub-Q Tissue

ORALS
Can the patient follow directions?
Can the patient swallow?

TOPICALS
Rectal
Sublingual
Nasal
Eyes
Ears
Transdermal

FORMS

INHALATION
MDI DPI Nebulizers

SOLIDS
Capsules - Pills
Tablets
Suppositories
Ointments & Powders

TRANSDERMAL

SOLUTIONS
Emulsions
Spirits
Syrups
Elixirs
Suspensions
Lotions

NURSING RESPONSIBILITIES

- Administer only what YOU prepare
- Be familiar with med
  Desired response
  Side effects
  Average dose
  Safety precautions
- Document meds
- Evaluate
  Patient's condition
  Med compatibility
  Allergies
- Aseptic technique
- Hand hygiene after removing gloves & between patients
- Review med administration if client is to do by himself

CJMILLER

Safe Administration

- Double check calculated doses with another RN.
- Call practitioner if dose is outside usual range.
- Check heparin, digoxin, insulin, chemo drugs with another RN prior to administration.

PEDS

Maximum safe dose based on child's weight =

Safe dose / Kg × Child's wt. in Kg

MED CALCULATIONS

ORAL

$$\frac{Dose\ Ordered}{Dose\ on\ Hand} = Amt.\ to\ give$$

$$\frac{Dose\ Ordered}{Dose\ on\ Hand} \times Quantity = Amt.\ to\ give$$

PARENTERAL

$$\frac{Dose\ Ordered}{Dose\ on\ Hand} \times Qty\ of\ Sol = Amt.\ to\ give\ (mLs)$$

IV

Drop "gtt" factor

Total mLs $$\frac{Total\ mLs}{x's\ Minutes} = mL \times gtt\ factor = gtt\ /\ min$$

$$\frac{mL\ /\ Hour}{60} = mL\ /\ min$$

$$\frac{Amt.\ to\ infuse}{Hour\ rate} = \#\ of\ hours$$

$$\frac{Amt.\ to\ infuse}{Infusion\ time} = mL\ /\ Hour$$

TIP – Estimate the answer in your mind – need to give 35mg – available 50mg in 5mL – you know your answer is less than 5mL, but over 2.5 mL.

ATROPINE OVERDOSE

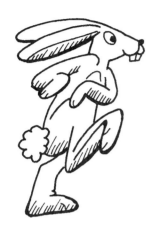

Hot as a Hare
(decreased sweating = ↑ temperature)

Mad as a Hatter
(confusion, delirium)

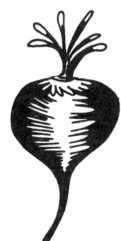

Red as a Beet
(flushed face)

Dry as a Bone
(decreased secretions, thirsty)

From: Robert W. Malone, RN

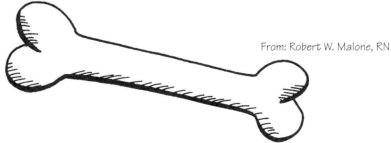

EAR DROPS ADMINISTRATION

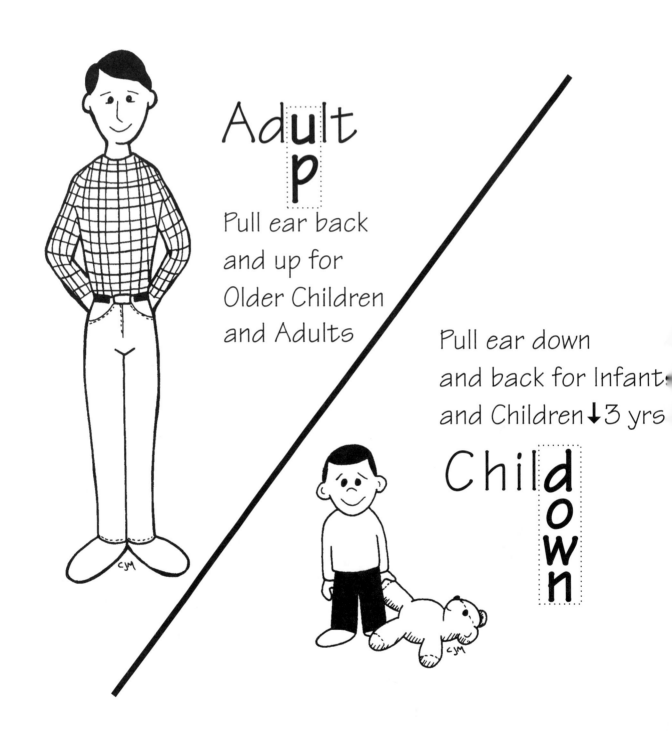

Adult
up

Pull ear back
and up for
Older Children
and Adults

Pull ear down
and back for Infant
and Children ↓3 yrs

Chil**down**

©Nursing Education Consultants, Inc.

Pharmacology
NursingEd.com

© 2012 Nursing Educat
Consultants,

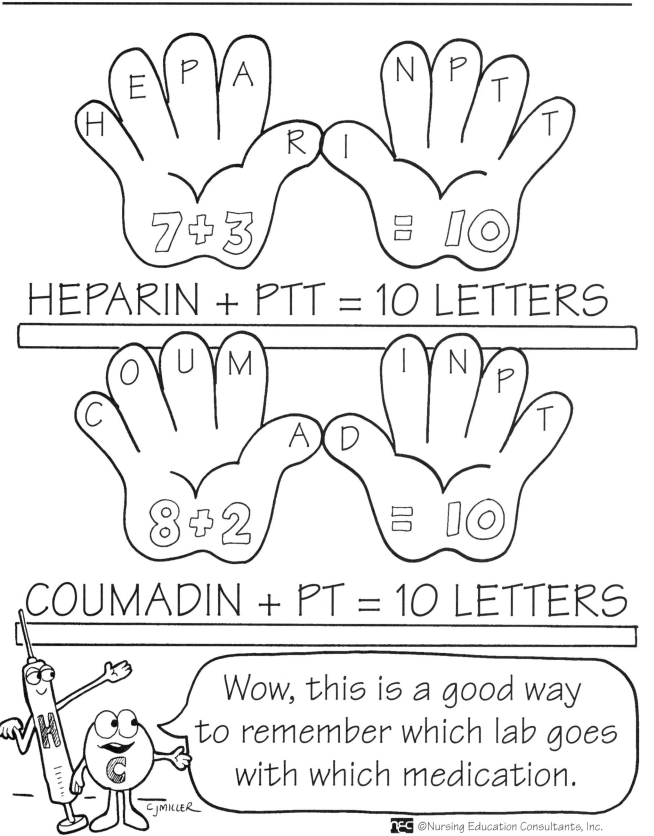

HEPARIN + PTT = 10 LETTERS

COUMADIN + PT = 10 LETTERS

Wow, this is a good way to remember which lab goes with which medication.

INFLAMMATION

H	**H**eat
I	**I**nduration
P	**P**ain
E	**E**dema
R	**R**edness

Adapted from Dolores Graceffa, RN, MS

Fluids, Acid-Base and Electrolytes
NursingEd.com

RESPIRATORY ACIDOSIS

- Hypoventilation → Hypoxia

- Rapid, Shallow Respirations

- $\downarrow$ BP

Skin/Mucosa Pale to Cyanotic

- Headache

- Hyperkalemia

- Dysrhythmias ($\uparrow K^+$)

- Drowsiness, Dizziness, Disorientation

I can't catch my breath.

- Muscle Weakness, Hyperreflexia

- Causes:
  Respiratory Depression (Anesthesia, Overdose, $\uparrow$ICP)
  Airway Obstruction
  $\downarrow$Alveolar Capillary Diffusion (Pneumonia, COPD, ARDS, PE)

$\downarrow$pH ($\downarrow$ 7.35) $\uparrow$PCO$_2$ ($\uparrow$48mmHg)

Retention of CO$_2$ by Lungs

CJMILLER

METABOLIC ACIDOSIS

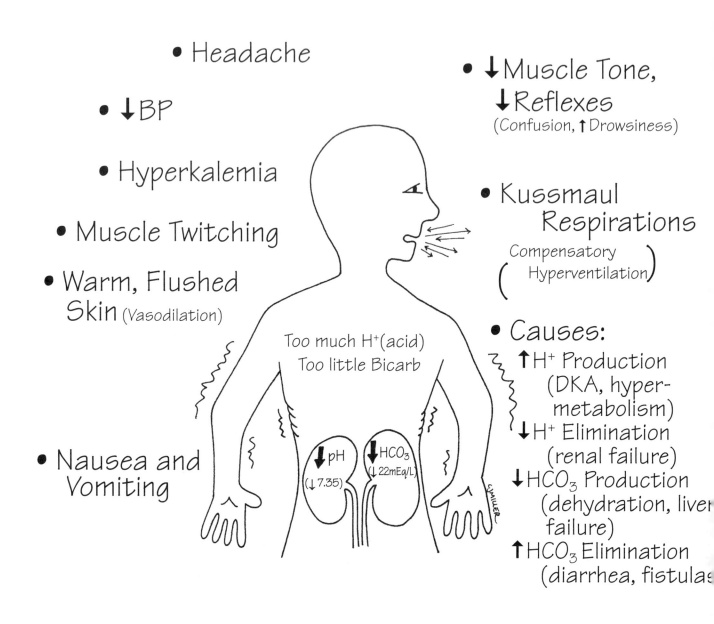

- Headache

- ↓BP

- Hyperkalemia

- Muscle Twitching

- Warm, Flushed Skin (Vasodilation)

- Nausea and Vomiting

- ↓Muscle Tone, ↓Reflexes (Confusion, ↑Drowsiness)

- Kussmaul Respirations
  Compensatory Hyperventilation)

- Causes:
  ↑H⁺ Production (DKA, hyper-metabolism)
  ↓H⁺ Elimination (renal failure)
  ↓HCO₃ Production (dehydration, liver failure)
  ↑HCO₃ Elimination (diarrhea, fistulas

Too much H⁺(acid)
Too little Bicarb

↓pH (↓7.35)   ↓HCO₃ (↓22mEq/L)

Fluids, Acid-Base and Electrolytes
NursingEd.com

© 2012 Nursing Educat
Consultants,

RESPIRATORY ALKALOSIS

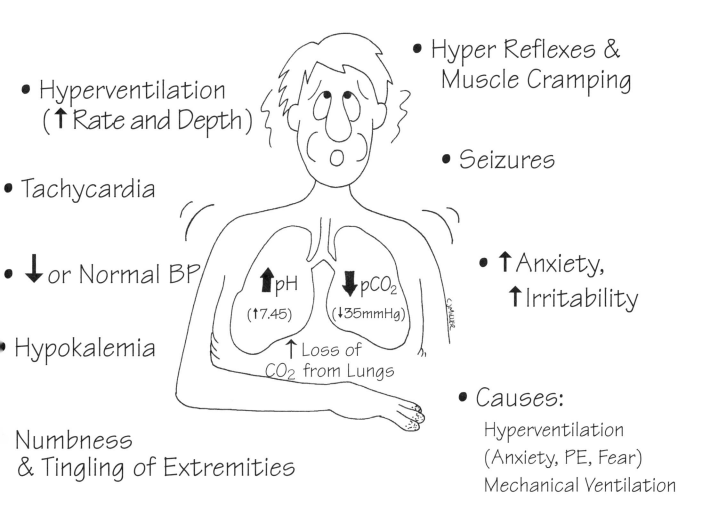

- Hyper Reflexes & Muscle Cramping

- Hyperventilation (↑Rate and Depth)

- Seizures

- Tachycardia

- ↓or Normal BP

↑pH (↑7.45)   ↓pCO₂ (↓35mmHg)

↑ Loss of CO₂ from Lungs

- ↑Anxiety, ↑Irritability

- Hypokalemia

Numbness & Tingling of Extremities

- Causes:
  Hyperventilation (Anxiety, PE, Fear)
  Mechanical Ventilation

©Nursing Education Consultants, Inc.

METABOLIC ALKALOSIS

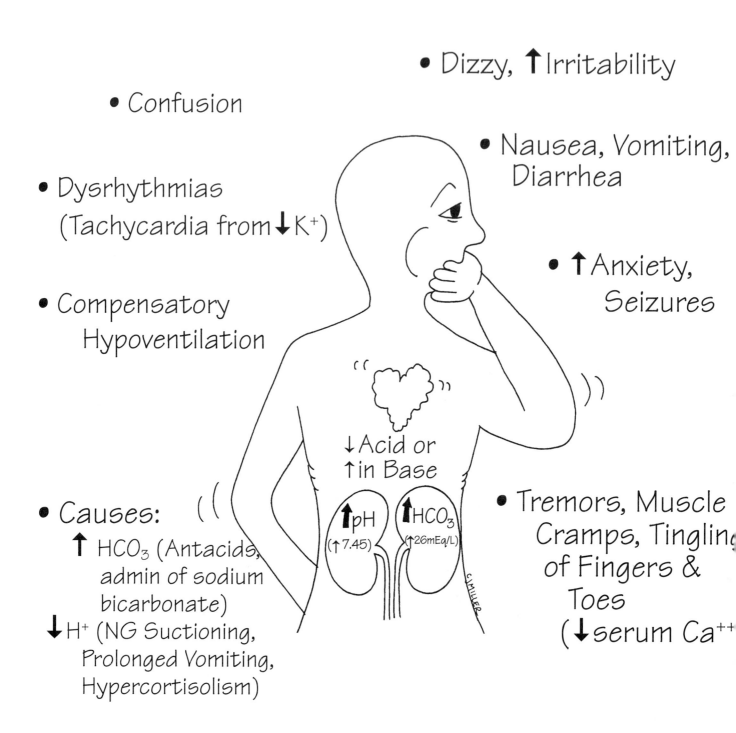

- Dizzy, ↑Irritability

- Confusion

- Nausea, Vomiting, Diarrhea

- Dysrhythmias (Tachycardia from ↓K⁺)

- ↑Anxiety, Seizures

- Compensatory Hypoventilation

↓Acid or ↑in Base

↑pH (↑7.45) ↑HCO₃ (↑26mEq/L)

- Causes:
  ↑ HCO₃ (Antacids, admin of sodium bicarbonate)
  ↓H⁺ (NG Suctioning, Prolonged Vomiting, Hypercortisolism)

- Tremors, Muscle Cramps, Tingling of Fingers & Toes (↓serum Ca⁺⁺

C.MILLER

Fluids, Acid-Base and Electrolytes
NursingEd.com

© 2012 Nursing Education Consultants, Inc

ACID BASE MNEMONIC
(ROME)

 Respiratory

Opposite

 pH $\uparrow$ PCO$_2$ $\downarrow$ Alkalosis

pH $\downarrow$ PCO$_2$ $\uparrow$ Acidosis

 Metabolic

Equal

 pH $\uparrow$ HCO$_3$ $\uparrow$ Alkalosis

pH $\downarrow$ HCO$_3$ $\downarrow$ Acidosis

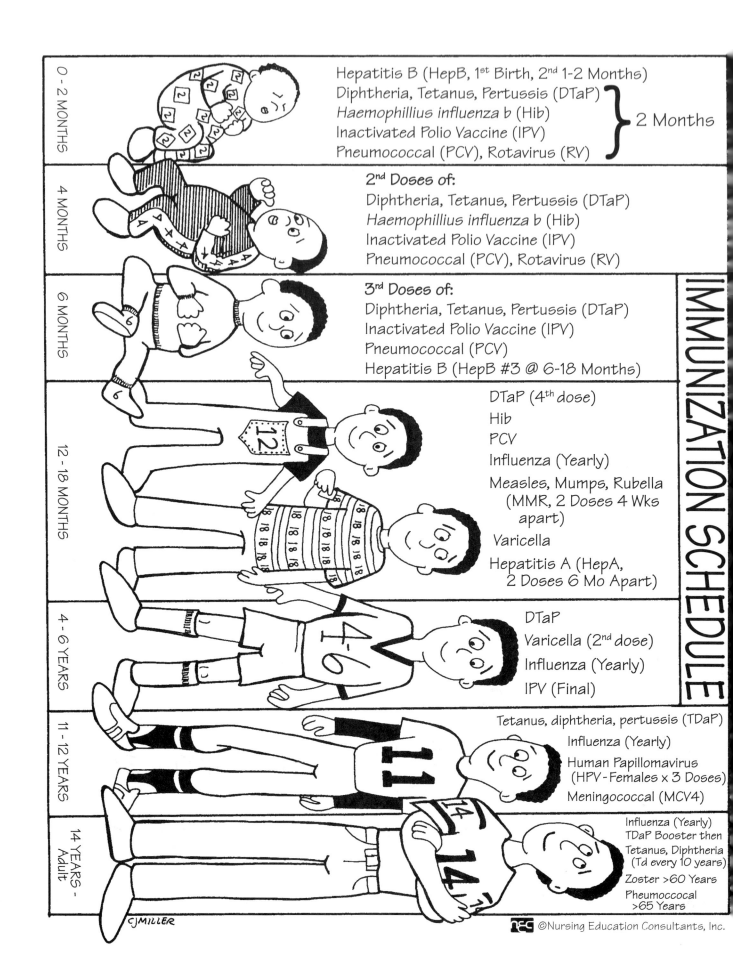

IMMUNIZATION SCHEDULE

0 - 2 MONTHS
Hepatitis B (HepB, 1st Birth, 2nd 1-2 Months)
Diphtheria, Tetanus, Pertussis (DTaP)
Haemophillius influenza b (Hib)
Inactivated Polio Vaccine (IPV)
Pneumococcal (PCV), Rotavirus (RV)
} 2 Months

4 MONTHS
2nd Doses of:
Diphtheria, Tetanus, Pertussis (DTaP)
Haemophillius influenza b (Hib)
Inactivated Polio Vaccine (IPV)
Pneumococcal (PCV), Rotavirus (RV)

6 MONTHS
3rd Doses of:
Diphtheria, Tetanus, Pertussis (DTaP)
Inactivated Polio Vaccine (IPV)
Pneumococcal (PCV)
Hepatitis B (HepB #3 @ 6-18 Months)

12 - 18 MONTHS
DTaP (4th dose)
Hib
PCV
Influenza (Yearly)
Measles, Mumps, Rubella
(MMR, 2 Doses 4 Wks apart)
Varicella
Hepatitis A (HepA, 2 Doses 6 Mo Apart)

4 - 6 YEARS
DTaP
Varicella (2nd dose)
Influenza (Yearly)
IPV (Final)

11 - 12 YEARS
Tetanus, diphtheria, pertussis (TDaP)
Influenza (Yearly)
Human Papillomavirus
(HPV - Females x 3 Doses)
Meningococcal (MCV4)

14 YEARS - Adult
Influenza (Yearly)
TDaP Booster then
Tetanus, Diphtheria
(Td every 10 years)
Zoster >60 Years
Pheumoccocal >65 Years

CJMILLER

Immune
NursingEd.com

HUMAN IMMUNODEFICIENCY VIRUS (HIV) INFECTION

Transmission:

- Unprotected Sexual Intercourse
- Contact with Blood and Blood Products
- Perinatal - during pregnancy, delivery, or breastfeeding

Screening:

- Enzyme immunoassay (EIA) at 3 wks, 6 wks, 3 mo after exposure
- Rapid HIV Antibody Testing — tests for antigens, not antibodies, if positive, need follow-up with EIA and/or Antibody/Antigen test

Seroconversion — development of HIV specific antibodies

- Window Period - may be 2 months between infection and detection of antibodies (HIV positive)

Acquired Immunodeficiency Disease Syndrome — (AIDS) presence of at least one or more:

- CD4 Tcell count ↓ 200 cells/uL (compromised immune system)
- Opportunistic infections —
  Fungal — Candidiasis, Pneumocystis jiroveci pneumonia (PCP)
  Viral — Cytomegalovirus (CMV)
  Bacterial — Mycobacterium tuberculosis, pneumonia
  Protozoal — Toxoplasmosis of brain, intestine
- Cancer
  Invasive cervical
  Kaposi's sarcoma
  Lymphoma
- Wasting Syndrome
- AIDS Dementia Complex

Early Chronic Infection

- HIV infection to development of AIDs — average 11 years
- Symptoms — fatigue, headache, lymphadenopathy, low grade fever
- Normal CD4$^+$ T-Cell count
- Increased infections

Intermediate Chronic Infection

- CD4$^+$ T-Cell count ↓ 200-500 cells/uL
- Increased viral load
- Increased infections, earlier symptoms more severe

Late Chronic Infection

- Diagnosis of AIDS

Treatment:

- Antiretroviral therapy (ART) begins with confirmation of HIV

Goals:

- Decrease viral load
- Maintain or ↑ CD4$^+$ T-Cell count
- Delay onset of HIV related symptoms
- Prevent or delay opportunistic infections

CJMILLER

©Nursing Education Consultants, Inc.

PREVENTION OF INFECTION

*Safe Injection Practices

- Use a Single Dose Syringe and Needle 1 Time and Discard
  - Do **NOT** Recap a Needle
  - Discard in Sharps Container
  - Do **NOT** Force a Syringe into a Full Sharps Container

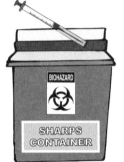

- Do **NOT** Place a Syringe and Needle –
  in your pocket
  on bedside table
  on a meal tray

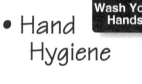

- Hand Hygiene

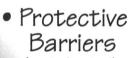

- Protective Barriers (as indicated)
  - Gloves
  - Mask
  - Eye Shield
  - Gown

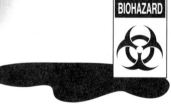

Maintain Standard Precautions

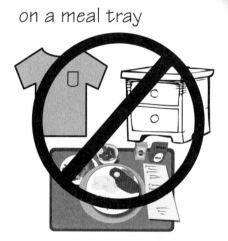

* Clean Up Spills of Body Fluids Immediately, Then Cleanse Area with Germicidal Solution.

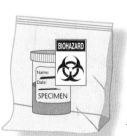

* Consider ALL Body Fluids to be Contaminated.

* Avoid Contaminating the Outside of Specimen Containers.

Immune
NursingEd.com

INFECTIOUS MONONUCLEOSIS
"Mono"

Transmission:
Most common in young people
↓25 yrs old
Predominantly transmitted via saliva.
Known as the "Kissing Disease"

Cause:
Epstein Barr Virus
(EBV)

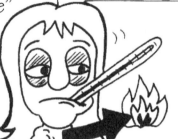

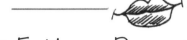

- Fatigue, Decreased Energy

Sore Throat (severe)

- Fever

- Tonsils Enlarged and Reddened

- Headache

- Skin Rash

- Swollen Lymph Glands

- Pain in LUQ – Splenomegaly

- Loss of Appetite

NEC ©Nursing Education Consultants, Inc.

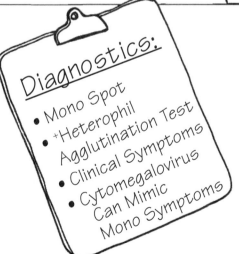

Diagnostics:
- Mono Spot
- +Heterophil Agglutination Test
- Clinical Symptoms
- Cytomegalovirus Can Mimic Mono Symptoms

Treatment:

- Rest
- Throat Soothing Measures
- Acetaminophen / Ibuprofen
- Low Energy / Impact Activity
- Gradual ↑Activity
- Course is Self-limiting

CAUTION
EARLY WARNING SIGNS

C **C**hange in bowel or bladder

A **A** lesion that does not heal

U **U**nexplained weight loss, fever, bleeding or discharg

T **T**hickening or lump in breast or elsewhere

I **I**ndigestion or difficulty swallowing

O **O**bvious changes in skin, wart or mole

N **N**agging pain, cough or persistent hoarsenes

Abnormal Cell Growth
NursingEd.com

CANCER

C   Comfort

A   Altered Body Image

N   Nutrition

C   Chemotherapy

E   Evaluate Response to Meds

R   Respite for Caretakers

©Nursing Education Consultants, Inc.

ALTERATIONS OF BODY IMAGE

IMPACT, SHOCK, DENIAL
Despair
Discouragement
Withdrawal

ANGER
Refusal to discuss
  change or loss
↓Self Esteem
Hostile / Irritable

DEPRESSION
Insomnia
Refusal to participate in self-care
Sadness

ADJUSTMENT
Acceptance and adaption
Active participant in
  therapy / care
Planning for future
↑Self-esteem

C.J. MILLER

GRIEF
Normal reaction to loss
Regression can and does occur
Provide safe environment for
  expression of feelings
Common in patients who have experi-
enced mastectomy, amputation,
burns, cancer, disfiguring surgery, or
spinal cord injury

©Nursing Education Consultants, Inc.

Psychosocial Nursing Concepts
NursingEd.com

BASIC COMPONENTS
OF A PSYCH ASSESSMENT

GENERAL HISTORY OF PATIENT

Name
Ethnicity
Marital Status
Living Arrangements
Occupation
Education
Cultural Implications
Religious & Spiritual
Beliefs/Affiliations

PRESENTING PROBLEM

Why is Patient
Seeking help?

Recent Difficulties

Relevant Family History

↑ Feelings of - Depression
                Anxiety
                Hopelessness
                Confusion
                Suspiciousness
                Being Overwhelmed

Somatic Changes

RELEVANT PERSONAL HISTORY

Previous Illness
and Hospitalizations

Growth and
Development Patterns

Social Patterns - Family
& Friends

Sexual Preference/Practice

Interests

Substance Use & Abuse

Coping Abilities

RELEVANT FAMILY HISTORY

Childhood

Adolescence

Drug Use

Physical, Emotional
or Sexual Abuse

Family Physical
or
Psychosocial
Problems

CJMILLER

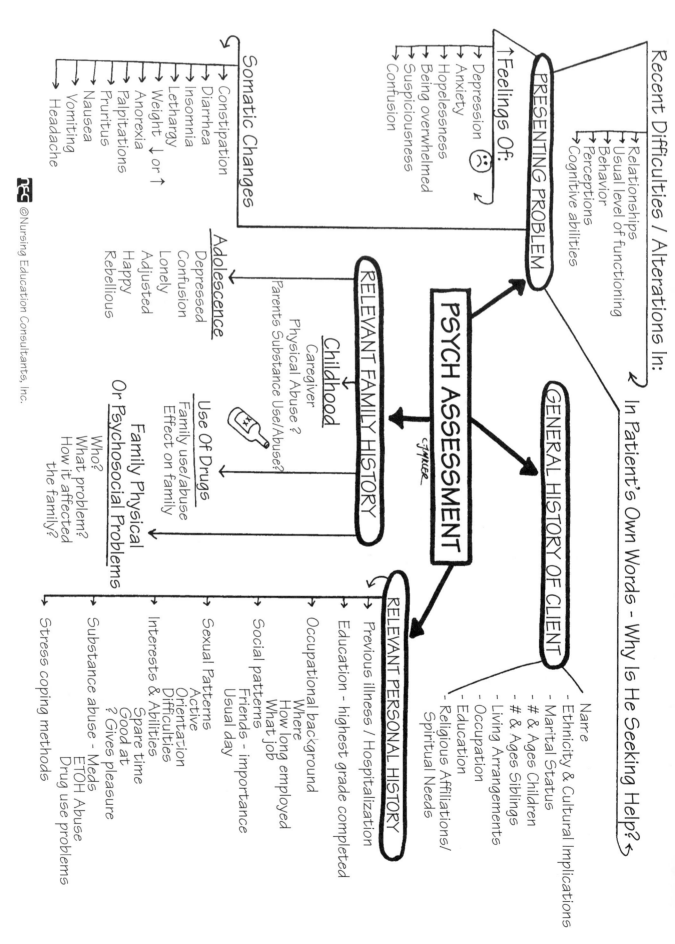

Recent Difficulties / Alterations In:
→ Relationships
→ Usual level of functioning
→ Behavior
→ Perceptions
→ Cognitive abilities

In Patient's Own Words - Why Is He Seeking Help?

PRESENTING PROBLEM

→Feelings Of:
→ Depression
→ Anxiety
→ Hopelessness
→ Being overwhelmed
→ Suspiciousness
→ Confusion

Somatic Changes
→ Constipation
→ Diarrhea
→ Insomnia
→ Lethargy
→ Weight ↓ or ↑
→ Anorexia
→ Palpitations
→ Pruritus
→ Nausea
→ Vomiting
→ Headache

PSYCH ASSESSMENT
JMiller

RELEVANT FAMILY HISTORY

Adolescence
Depressed
Confusion
Lonely
Adjusted
Happy
Rebellious

Childhood
Caregiver
Physical Abuse ?
Parents Substance Use/Abuse?

Use Of Drugs
Family use/abuse
Effect on family

Family Physical
Or Psychosocial Problems
Who?
What problem?
How it affected
the family?

GENERAL HISTORY OF CLIENT
- Name
- Ethnicity & Cultural Implications
- Marital Status
- # & Ages Children
- # & Ages Siblings
- Living Arrangements
- Occupation
- Education
- Religious Affiliations/
  Spiritual Needs

RELEVANT PERSONAL HISTORY
→ Previous Illness / Hospitalization
→ Education - highest grade completed
→ Occupational background
   Where
   How long employed
   What job
→ Social patterns
   Friends - importance
   Usual day
→ Sexual Patterns
   Active
   Orientation
   Difficulties
→ Interests & Abilities
   Spare time
   Good at
   ? Gives pleasure
→ Substance abuse - Meds
   ETOH Abuse
   Drug use problems
→ Stress coping methods

Psychosocial Nursing Concepts
NursingEd.com

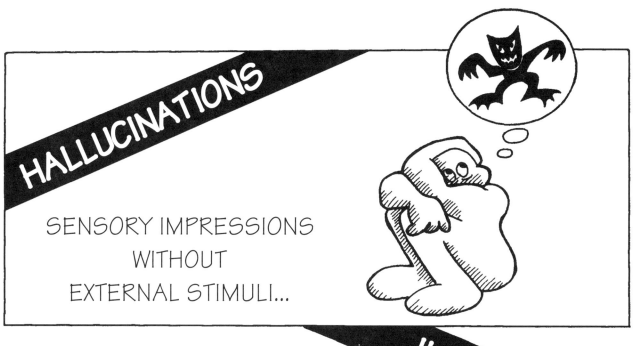

HALLUCINATIONS

SENSORY IMPRESSIONS
WITHOUT
EXTERNAL STIMULI...

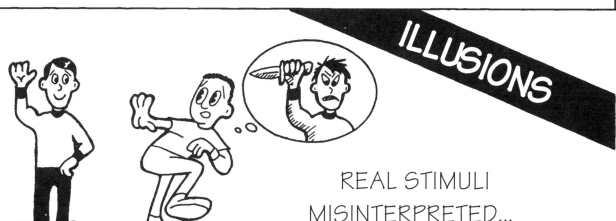

ILLUSIONS

REAL STIMULI
MISINTERPRETED...

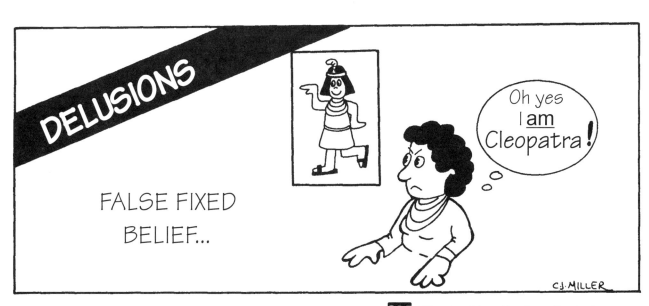

DELUSIONS

FALSE FIXED
BELIEF...

MENTAL RETARDATION

R **R**outine

R **R**epetition

R **R**einforcement

R **R**outine

R **R**epetition

R **R**einforcement

R **R**outine

R **R**epetition

R **R**einforcement

ALCOHOL WITHDRAWAL DELIRIUM
"Delirium Tremens (DTs)"

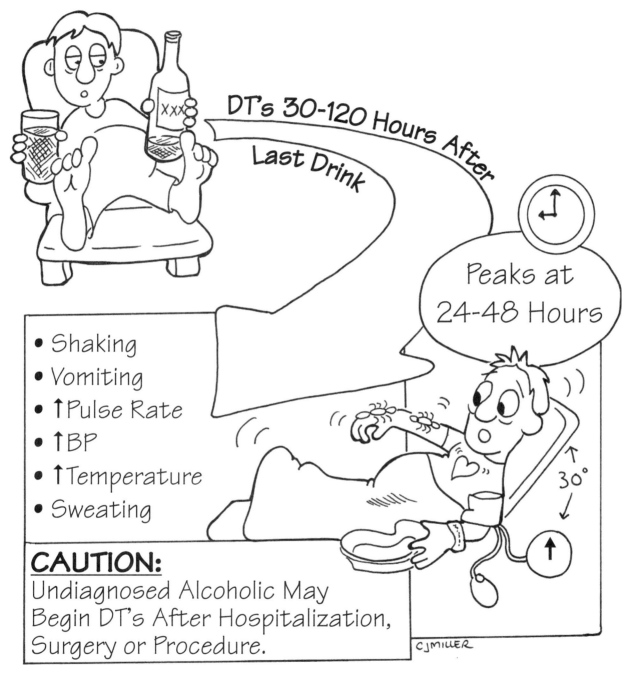

DT's 30-120 Hours After Last Drink

Peaks at 24-48 Hours

- Shaking
- Vomiting
- ↑Pulse Rate
- ↑BP
- ↑Temperature
- Sweating

CAUTION:
Undiagnosed Alcoholic May Begin DT's After Hospitalization, Surgery or Procedure.

CJMILLER

©Nursing Education Consultants, Inc.

ASSESS CHANGES IN SENILE DEMENTIA

J   **J**udgment

A   **A**ffect

M   **M**emory

C   **C**ognition

O   **O**rientation

©Nursing Education Consultants, Inc.

EATING DISORDERS

ANOREXIA NERVOSA

Views self as fat – regardless of weight

Intense fear of becoming fat

Anxious about losing control

Weight is ↓85% of normal

Feels powerless

Associated with obsessive compulsive disorder

BULIMIA

Recurrent binge eating followed by

self-induced vomiting, misuse of laxatives and enemas

Depressed mood following binge eating

↑Anxiety and compulsivity

PICA

Persistent eating of non-nutritive food and non-food substances

Food – cornstarch, baking powder, coffee grounds

Non-food – clay, soils, laundry starch paint chips

More common in children, pregnant women, individuals with autism or cognitive impairment, patients in chronic renal failure.

Influenced by cultural background.

Associated with iron and zinc deficiency.

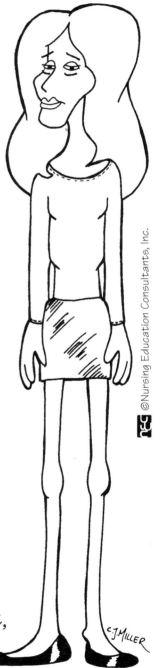

©Nursing Education Consultants, Inc.

c.j.Miller

BIPOLAR DISORDER

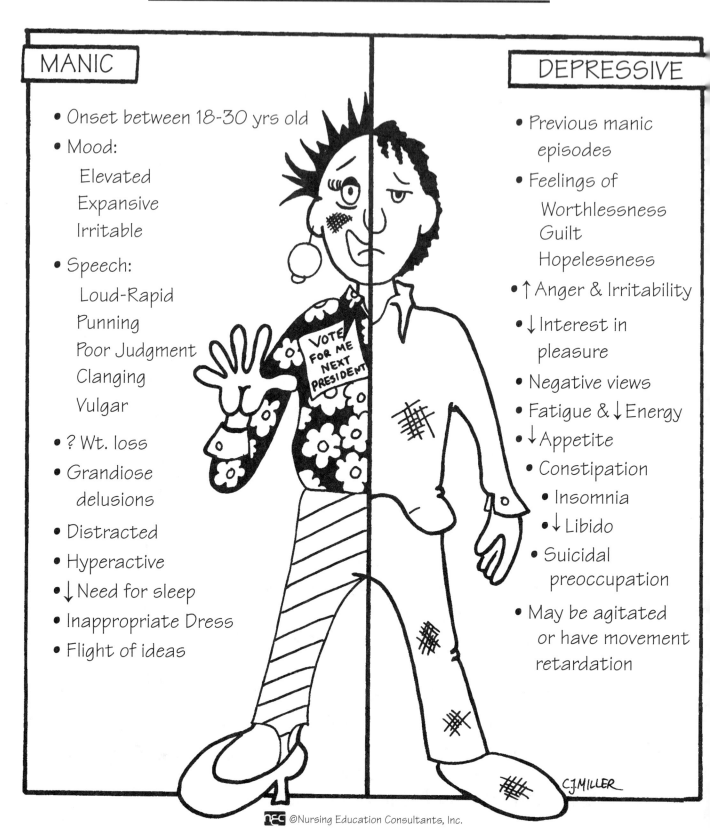

MANIC

- Onset between 18-30 yrs old
- Mood:
    Elevated
    Expansive
    Irritable
- Speech:
    Loud-Rapid
    Punning
    Poor Judgment
    Clanging
    Vulgar
- ? Wt. loss
- Grandiose
    delusions
- Distracted
- Hyperactive
- ↓ Need for sleep
- Inappropriate Dress
- Flight of ideas

DEPRESSIVE

- Previous manic
    episodes
- Feelings of
    Worthlessness
    Guilt
    Hopelessness
- ↑ Anger & Irritability
- ↓ Interest in
    pleasure
- Negative views
- Fatigue & ↓ Energy
- ↓ Appetite
- Constipation
- Insomnia
- ↓ Libido
- Suicidal
    preoccupation
- May be agitated
    or have movement
    retardation

VOTE FOR ME NEXT PRESIDENT

CJ.MILLER

©Nursing Education Consultants, Inc.

Psychosocial Nursing Concepts
NursingEd.com

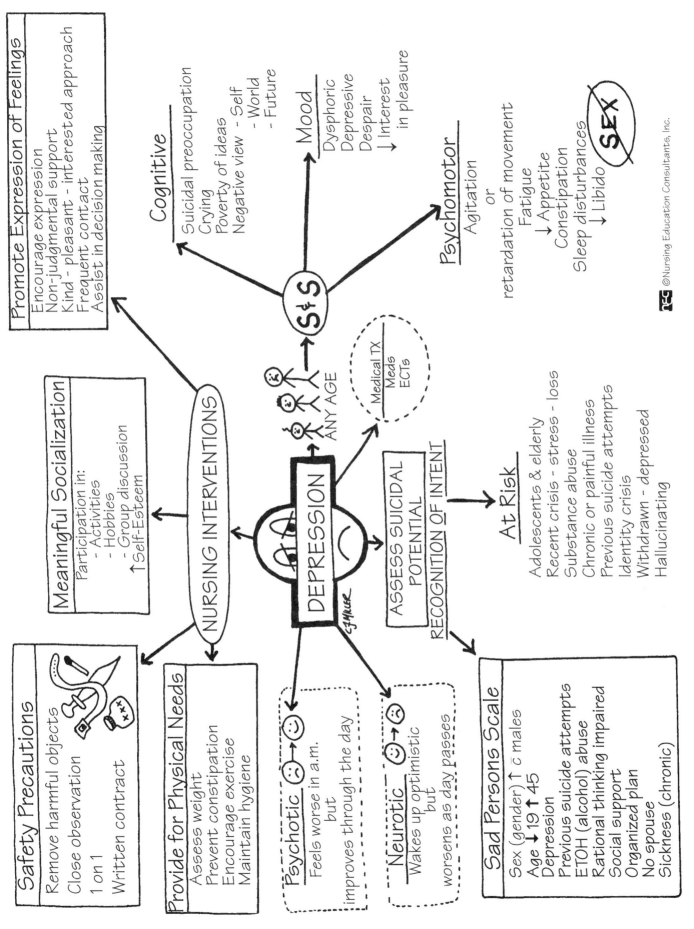

Promote Expression of Feelings
Encourage expression
Non-judgmental support
Kind - pleasant - interested approach
Frequent contact
Assist in decision making

Cognitive
Suicidal preoccupation
Crying
Poverty of ideas
Negative view - Self
- World
- Future

Mood
Dysphoric
Depressive
Despair
↓ Interest
in pleasure

Psychomotor
Agitation
or
retardation of movement
Fatigue
↓ Appetite
Constipation
Sleep disturbances
↓ Libido
~~SEX~~

S & S

ANY AGE

Medical TX
Meds
ECTs

Meaningful Socialization
Participation in:
- Activities
- Hobbies
- Group discussion
↑ Self-Esteem

NURSING INTERVENTIONS

DEPRESSION

ASSESS SUICIDAL POTENTIAL
RECOGNITION OF INTENT

At Risk
Adolescents & elderly
Recent crisis - stress - loss
Substance abuse
Chronic or painful illness
Previous suicide attempts
Identity crisis
Withdrawn - depressed
Hallucinating

Safety Precautions
Remove harmful objects
Close observation
1 on 1
Written contract

Provide for Physical Needs
Assess weight
Prevent constipation
Encourage exercise
Maintain hygiene

Psychotic ☹ → ☺
Feels worse in a.m.
but
improves through the day

Neurotic ☺ → ☹
Wakes up optimistic
but
worsens as day passes

Sad Persons Scale
Sex (gender) ↑ c̄ males
Age ↓ 19 ↑ 45
Depression
Previous suicide attempts
ETOH (alcohol) abuse
Rational thinking impaired
Social support
Organized plan
No spouse
Sickness (chronic)

SUICIDE PRECAUTIONS

SECURE ROOM:
- Windows Locked
- Breakproof Glass & Mirrors
- Plastic Flatware

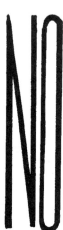

NO
- Cords - Phone
  - Extension
  - Equipment
  - Curtains
- Belts/Shoelaces/Drawstring Pants
- Matches or Cigarettes
- Sharps/Razors

PATIENT CARE:
- Frequent Observation... Preferably 1 to 1
- Staff Communication — Constant Risk Assessment/Documentatio
- Develop Therapeutic Relationship
- Written Behavior Contract with Pt.
- Restraints as Necessary
- Medications
- Monitor and Restrict Visitors

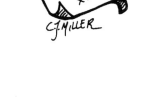

© 2012 Nursing Educatic
Consultants, In.

SCHIZOPHRENIA

- Illogical Thinking
    & Impaired Judgment
- Loss of Ego Boundaries
- Inability to Trust
- Bizarre Behavior
- Indifferent - Aloof
- Love/Hate Feelings
- Feelings of
    Rejection
    Lack of Self-Respect
    Loneliness, Hopelessness
- Speech Incoherent & Rambling
- Disorganized Thinking
- Autism

- Auditory Hallucinations
- Delusions – Persecutory
    or Grandiose
- Hypersensitivity to Sound,
    Sight & Smell
- Difficulty Relating to Others
- Negativism
- Religiosity
- Lack of Social Awareness
- Behavior – Disorganized, Motor
    Agitation, Catatonic
- Retreat to
    Fantasy World

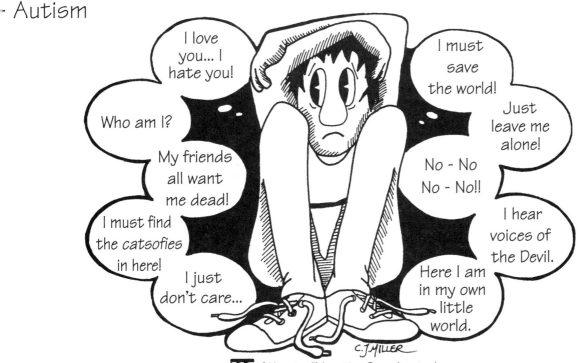

©Nursing Education Consultants, Inc.

EYE MEDICATIONS

MI<u>O</u>TIC

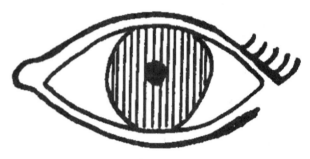

(Little Word - Little Pupil)

MY<u>D</u>RIATIC

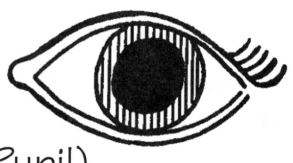

(Big Word - Big Pupil)

Do <u>not</u> give eye meds after using hand hygiene solution – ↑ eye irritation

Sensory
NursingEd.com

CATARACT

Characteristics

Cloudy, opaque lens

↓ Visual Acuity

No pain

Occurs gradually

↓ Night Vision

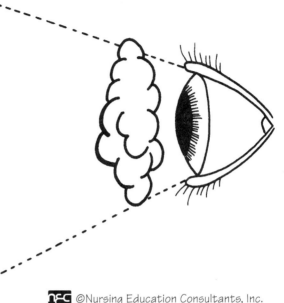

©Nursing Education Consultants, Inc.

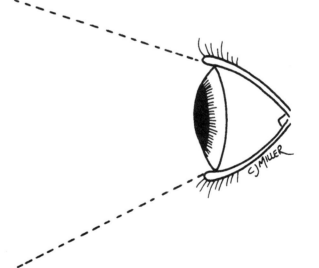

Treatment

Removal of lens with lens implant

HYPERTHYROIDISM

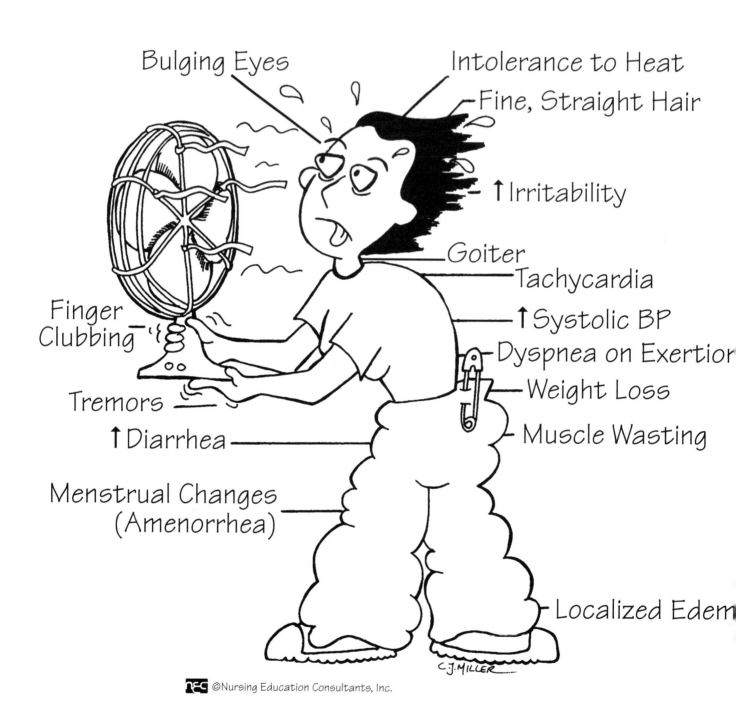

Bulging Eyes

Intolerance to Heat

Fine, Straight Hair

↑ Irritability

Goiter

Tachycardia

↑ Systolic BP

Dyspnea on Exertion

Weight Loss

Muscle Wasting

Finger Clubbing

Tremors

↑ Diarrhea

Menstrual Changes (Amenorrhea)

Localized Edem

C.J. MILLER

HYPOTHYROIDISM

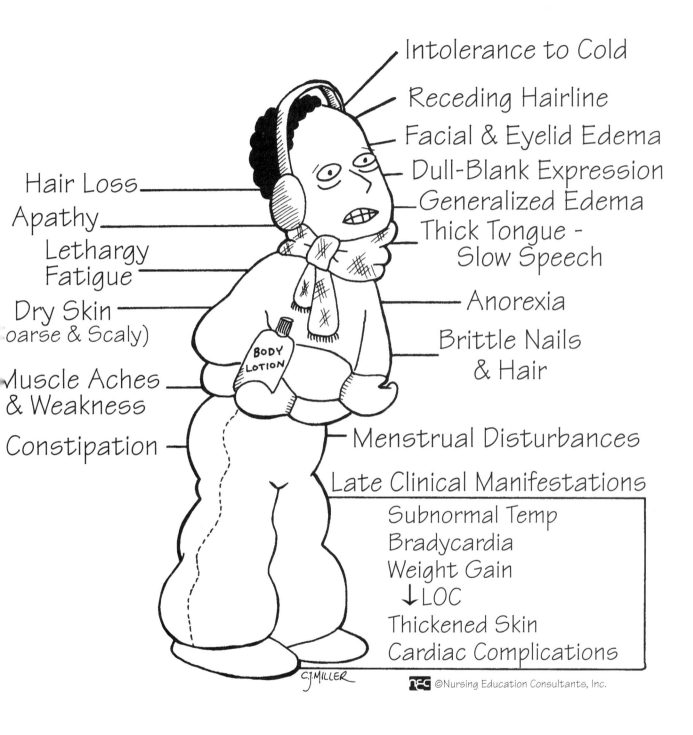

Intolerance to Cold

Receding Hairline

Facial & Eyelid Edema

Dull-Blank Expression

Generalized Edema

Thick Tongue -
Slow Speech

Hair Loss

Apathy

Lethargy
Fatigue

Dry Skin
(Coarse & Scaly)

Muscle Aches
& Weakness

Constipation

Anorexia

Brittle Nails
& Hair

Menstrual Disturbances

BODY LOTION

Late Clinical Manifestations

Subnormal Temp
Bradycardia
Weight Gain
↓LOC
Thickened Skin
Cardiac Complications

C.J.MILLER

©Nursing Education Consultants, Inc.

DIABETES INSIPIDUS (DI)

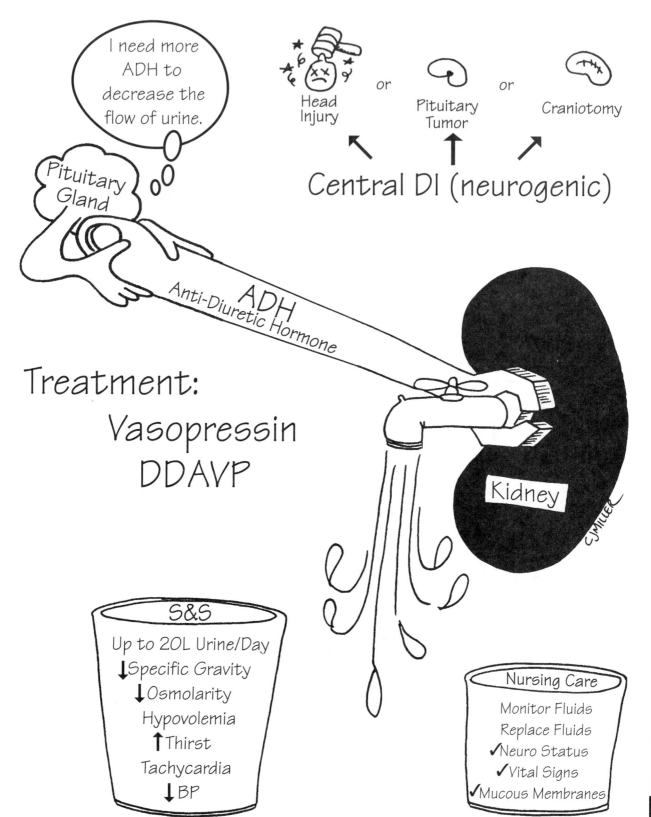

I need more ADH to decrease the flow of urine.

Pituitary Gland

Head Injury or Pituitary Tumor or Craniotomy

Central DI (neurogenic)

ADH
Anti-Diuretic Hormone

Treatment:
Vasopressin
DDAVP

Kidney

S&S
Up to 20L Urine/Day
↓Specific Gravity
↓Osmolarity
Hypovolemia
↑Thirst
Tachycardia
↓BP

Nursing Care
Monitor Fluids
Replace Fluids
✓Neuro Status
✓Vital Signs
✓Mucous Membranes

DIABETES MELLITUS - TYPE 1
SIGNS & SYMPTOMS:

Polyuria
↑Urination

Polydipsia
↑Thirst

Polyphagia
↑Hunger

- Weight Loss
- Fatigue
- ↑ Frequency of Infections
- Rapid Onset
- Insulin 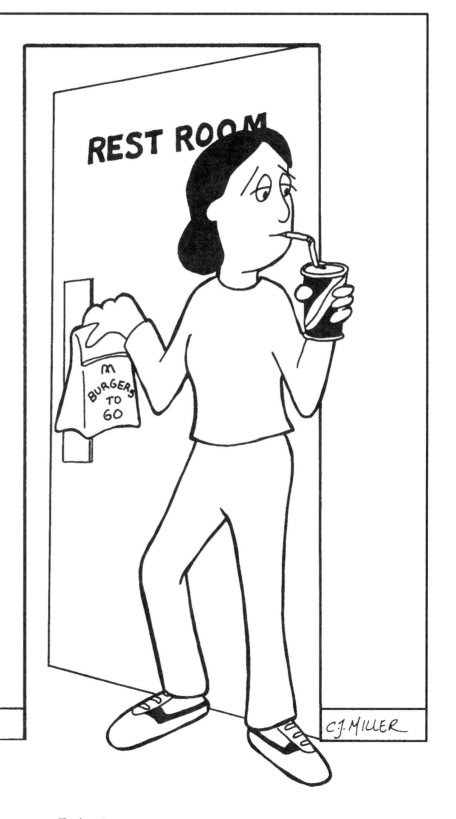 Dependent
- Familial Tendency
- Peak Incidence From 10 to 15 Years

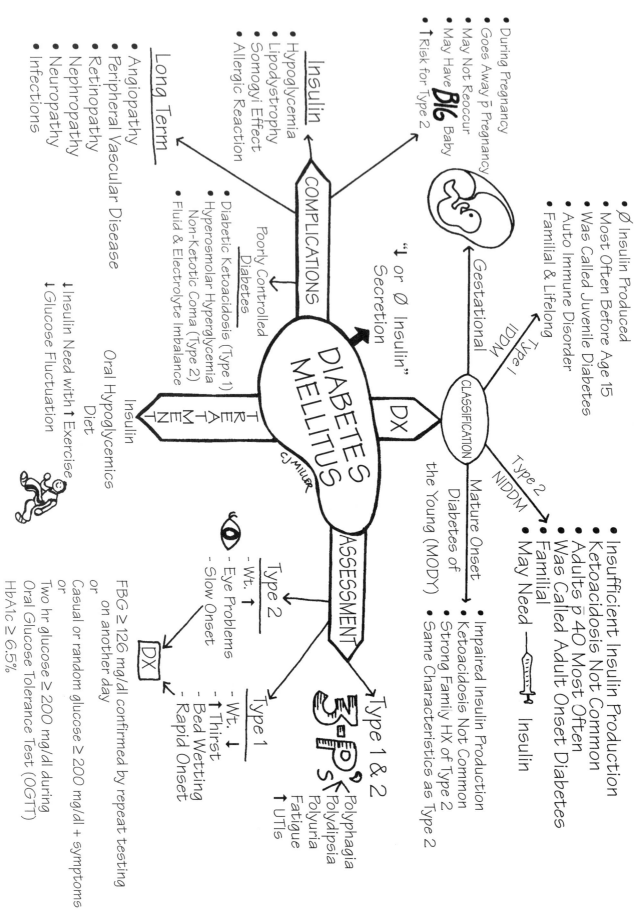

DIABETES MELLITUS

CJ Miller

"↓ or Ø Insulin" Secretion

CLASSIFICATION

Gestational
- During Pregnancy
- Goes Away p̄ Pregnancy
- May Not Reoccur
- May Have Big Baby
- ↑ Risk for Type 2

Type 1 / IDDM
- Ø Insulin Produced
- Most Often Before Age 15
- Was Called Juvenile Diabetes
- Auto Immune Disorder
- Familial & Lifelong

Type 2 / NIDDM
- Insufficient Insulin Production
- Ketoacidosis Not Common
- Adults p̄ 40 Most Often
- Was Called Adult Onset Diabetes
- Familial
- May Need Insulin

Mature Onset Diabetes of the Young (MODY)
- Impaired Insulin Production
- Ketoacidosis Not Common
- Strong Family HX of Type 2
- Same Characteristics as Type 2

COMPLICATIONS

Insulin
- Hypoglycemia
- Lipodystrophy
- Somogyi Effect
- Allergic Reaction

Poorly Controlled Diabetes
- Diabetic Ketoacidosis (Type 1)
- Hyperosmolar Hyperglycemia Non-Ketotic Coma (Type 2)
- Fluid & Electrolyte Imbalance

Long Term
- Angiopathy
- Peripheral Vascular Disease
- Retinopathy
- Nephropathy
- Neuropathy
- Infections

TREATMENT
- Insulin
- Oral Hypoglycemics
- Diet
- ↓ Insulin Need with ↑ Exercise
- ↑ Glucose Fluctuation

ASSESSMENT

Type 2
- Wt. ↑
- Eye Problems
- Slow Onset

Type 1
- Wt. ↓
- ↑ Thirst
- Bed Wetting
- Rapid Onset

3-P's
- Polyphagia
- Polydipsia
- Polyuria
- Fatigue
- ↑ UTIs

Type 1 & 2

DX

FBG ≥ 126 mg/dl confirmed by repeat testing on another day

or

Casual or random glucose ≥ 200 mg/dl during + symptoms

or

Two hr glucose ≥ 200 mg/dl during Oral Glucose Tolerance Test (OGTT)

HbA1c ≥ 6.5%

BLOOD SUGAR MNEMONIC

HOT & DRY = SUGAR HIGH

OLD & CLAMMY = NEED SOME CANDY

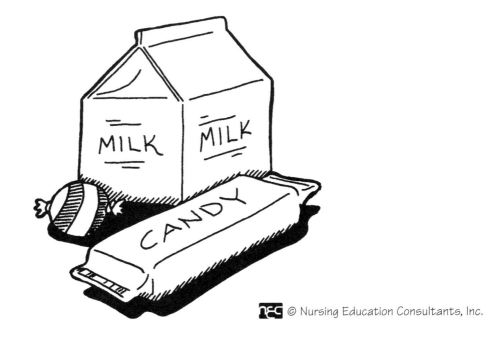

TRIANGLE OF
DIABETES MANAGEMENT

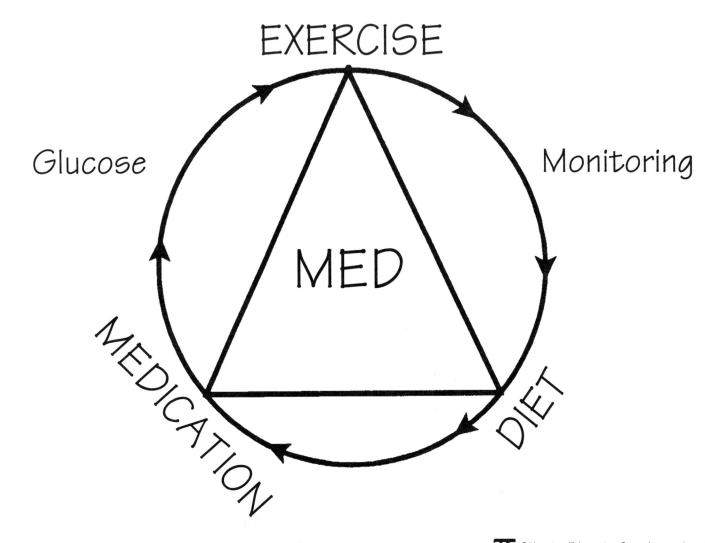

EXERCISE

Glucose

Monitoring

MED

MEDICATION

DIET

Endocrine
NursingEd.com

HYPOGLYCEMIA

T   Tachycardia

I   Irritable

R   Restless

E   Excessive Hunger

D   Diaphoresis
     Depression

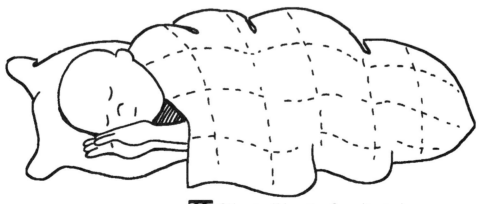

©Nursing Education Consultants, Inc.

METABOLIC SYNDROME - SYNDROME

Avoid the X Factor
Leads to: Diabetes, Stroke
and Heart Disease.

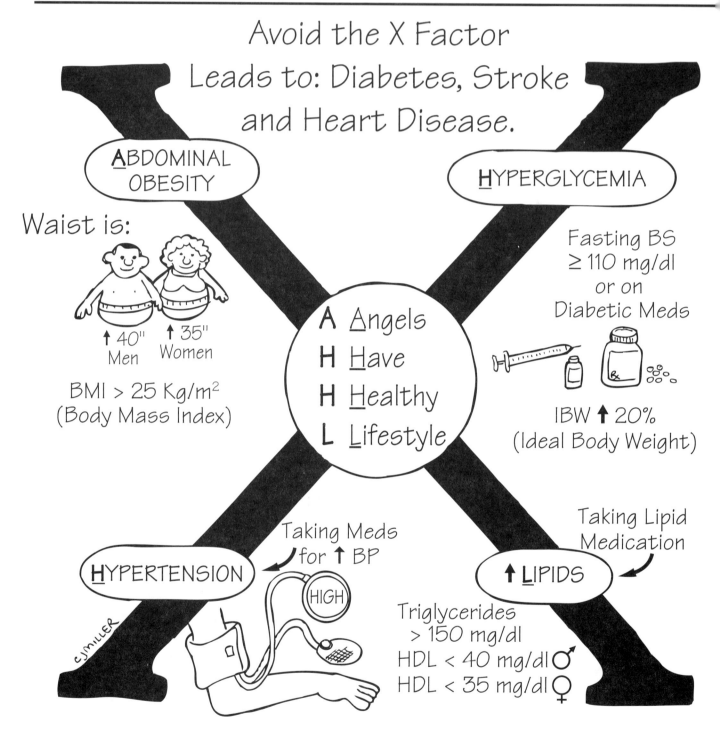

ABDOMINAL OBESITY

Waist is:

↑ 40" Men   ↑ 35" Women

BMI > 25 Kg/m² (Body Mass Index)

HYPERGLYCEMIA

Fasting BS ≥ 110 mg/dl or on Diabetic Meds

IBW ↑ 20% (Ideal Body Weight)

A **A**ngels
H **H**ave
H **H**ealthy
L **L**ifestyle

HYPERTENSION

Taking Meds for ↑ BP

HIGH

↑ LIPIDS

Taking Lipid Medication

Triglycerides > 150 mg/dl
HDL < 40 mg/dl ♂
HDL < 35 mg/dl ♀

ADDISON'S DISEASE
Adrenocortical Insufficiency

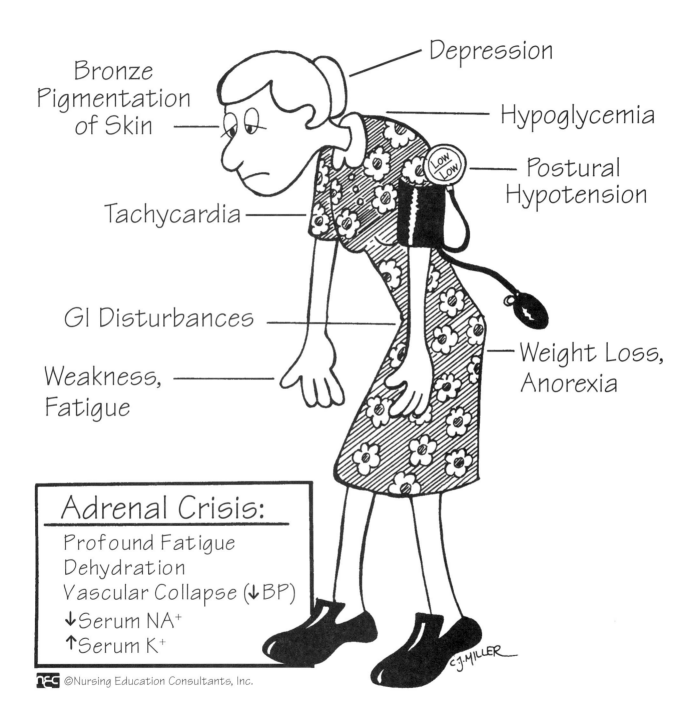

Depression

Bronze Pigmentation of Skin

Hypoglycemia

Postural Hypotension

Tachycardia

GI Disturbances

Weight Loss, Anorexia

Weakness, Fatigue

Low Low

Adrenal Crisis:
Profound Fatigue
Dehydration
Vascular Collapse ($\downarrow$BP)
$\downarrow$Serum NA$^+$
$\uparrow$Serum K$^+$

C.J.MILLER

CUSHING'S SYNDROME
Corticosteroid Excess

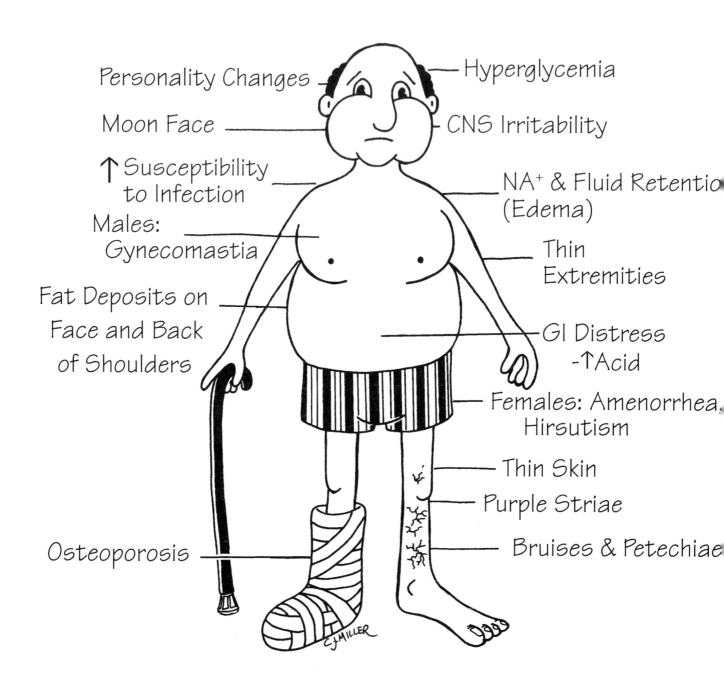

Personality Changes

Moon Face

↑ Susceptibility to Infection

Males: Gynecomastia

Fat Deposits on Face and Back of Shoulders

Osteoporosis

Hyperglycemia

CNS Irritability

NA⁺ & Fluid Retentio (Edema)

Thin Extremities

GI Distress -↑Acid

Females: Amenorrhea Hirsutism

Thin Skin

Purple Striae

Bruises & Petechiae

CJMILLER

ADRENAL GLAND HORMONES

S Sugar (Glucocorticoids)

S Salt (Mineralcorticoids)

S Sex (Androgens)

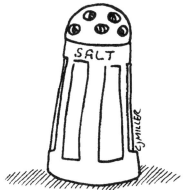

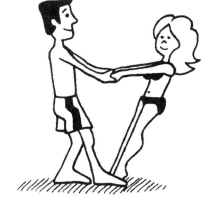

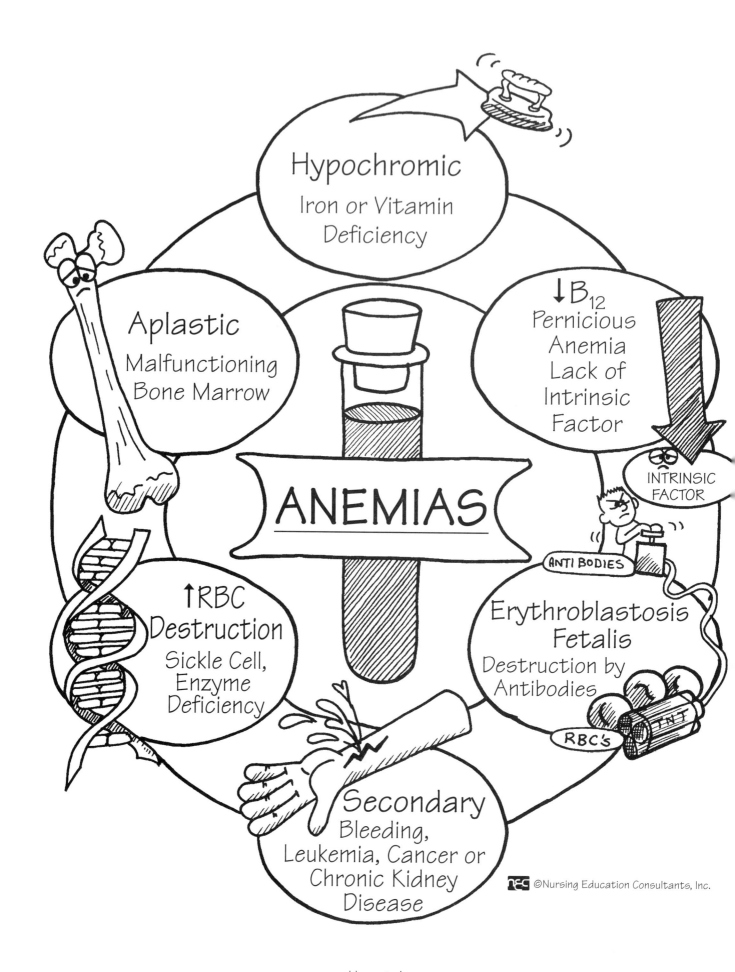

ANEMIAS

Hypochromic
Iron or Vitamin Deficiency

Aplastic
Malfunctioning Bone Marrow

↓B₁₂ Pernicious Anemia Lack of Intrinsic Factor

INTRINSIC FACTOR

ANTIBODIES

↑RBC Destruction
Sickle Cell, Enzyme Deficiency

Erythroblastosis Fetalis
Destruction by Antibodies

RBC's

TNT

Secondary
Bleeding, Leukemia, Cancer or Chronic Kidney Disease

©Nursing Education Consultants, Inc.

BLOOD ADMINISTRATION

* Determine Patient's
  • Allergies
  • Previous Transfusion
    Reactions

Administer Within 30 Minutes of
Receiving From Blood Bank

* Never Add **ANY** Meds
  to Blood Products

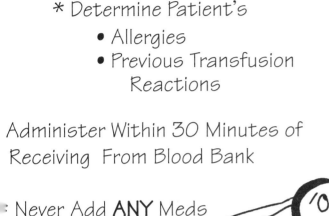

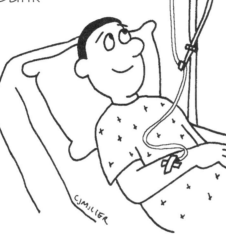

* Check Crossmatch
  Record With
  2 Nurses:
  • ABO-Group
  • RH Type
  • Patient's Name
  • ID Blood Band
  • Hospital #
  • Expiration Date

* Do **NOT** Warm Unless
  Risk of
  Hypothermic Response
  THEN Only By Specific
  Blood Warming Equipment

* Infuse Each Unit Over
  2-4 Hours **BUT**
  No Longer Than 4 Hours

KEY POINTS

- Verify Patient's ID
- Check the Dr's Order
- Check labels on blood bag &
  blood bank transfusion record
- Baseline vitals - (Then per policy)
- #18G or #20G gauge needle
- Normal saline IV solution
- Blood administration set with filter
- Severe reactions most likely
  first 15 min & first 50cc
- Blood tubing should be changed
  after 4 hours

@Nursing Education Consultants, Inc.

BLOOD TRANSFUSION REACTION

Febrile Reaction:
- Chills • Fever • Headache
- Flushing • Tachycardia • ↑ Anxiety

Allergic Reaction:
Mild:
- Hives • Pruritus
- Facial Flushing
Severe:
- Shortness of Breath
- Bronchospasm
- Anxiety

Hemolytic Transfusion Reaction:
- ↑ Anxiety
- Low Back Pain
- Hypotension
- Tachycardia
- Fever and Chills
- Chest Pain
- Tachypnea
- Hemoglobinuria
- May Have Immediate Onset

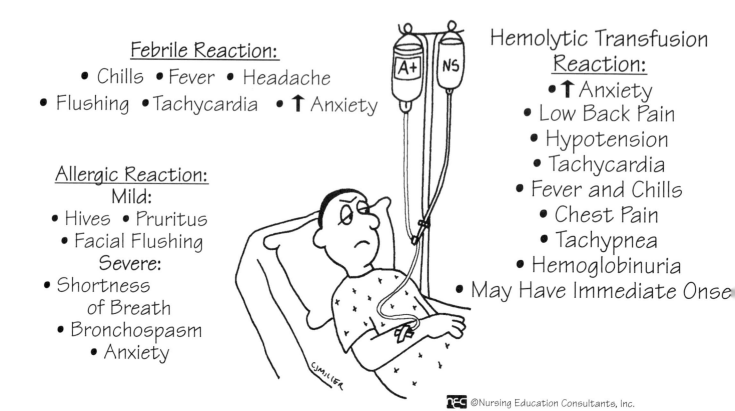

©Nursing Education Consultants, Inc.

⭐ Nursing Implications:
- Stop Transfusion and notify Physician
- Change IV tubing at hub and begin NS
- Treat symptoms if present→O_2, fluids, epinephrine
- Check vital signs every 15 minutes
- Recheck crossmatch record with unit and send blood bag/tubing to the lab
- Obtain blood sample
- Obtain urine sample for hemoglobinuria
- Monitor fluid/electrolyte balance
- Evaluate serum calcium levels

Hematology
NursingEd.com

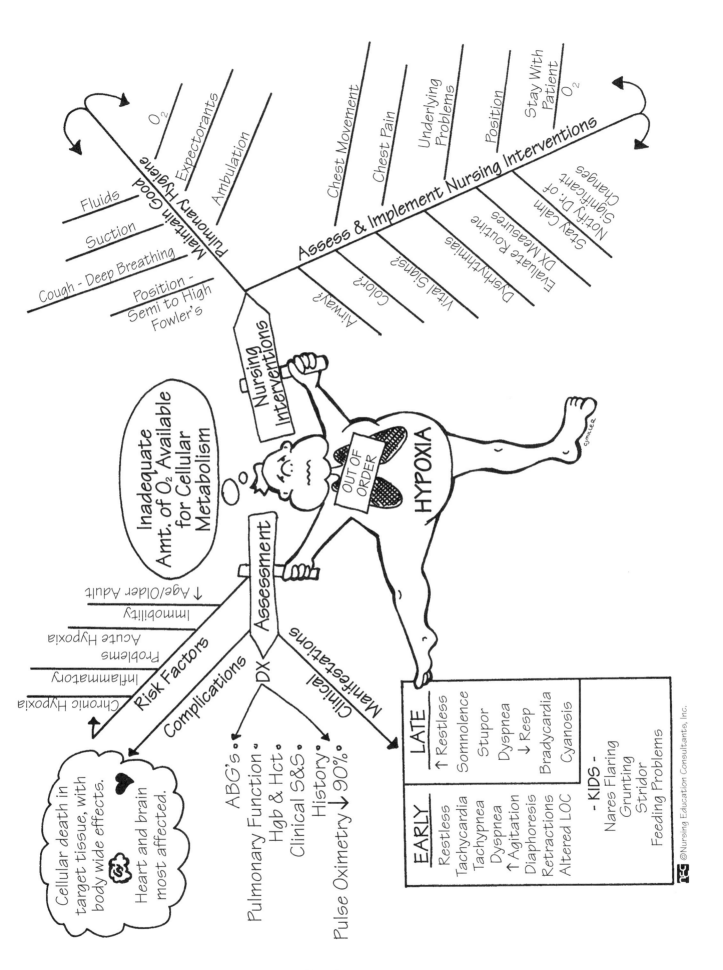

HYPOXIA

Inadequate Amt. of O_2 Available for Cellular Metabolism

Nursing Interventions

Maintain Good Pulmonary Hygiene
- O_2
- Expectorants
- Ambulation
- Fluids
- Suction
- Cough - Deep Breathing
- Position - Semi to High Fowler's

Assess & Implement Nursing Interventions
- Chest Movement
- Chest Pain
- Underlying Problems
- Position
- Stay With Patient
- O_2
- Airway?
- Color?
- Vital Signs?
- Dysrhythmias
- Evaluate Routine DX Measures
- Stay Calm
- Notify Dr. of Significant Changes

Assessment

Risk Factors
- ↑ Age/Older Adult
- Immobility
- Acute Hypoxia
- Inflammatory
- Chronic Hypoxia

Complications
- Cellular death in target tissue, with body wide effects.
- Heart and brain most affected.

DX
- ABG's
- Pulmonary Function - Hgb & Hct
- Clinical S&S
- History
- Pulse Oximetry ↓ 90%

Clinical Manifestations

EARLY
Restless
Tachycardia
Tachypnea
Dyspnea
↑ Agitation
Diaphoresis
Retractions
Altered LOC

LATE
↑ Restless
Somnolence
Stupor
Dyspnea
↓ Resp
Bradycardia
Cyanosis

- KIDS -
Nares Flaring
Grunting
Stridor
Feeding Problems

OUT OF ORDER

CMiller

©Nursing Education Consultants, Inc.

ASTHMA
(Reactive Airway Disease)

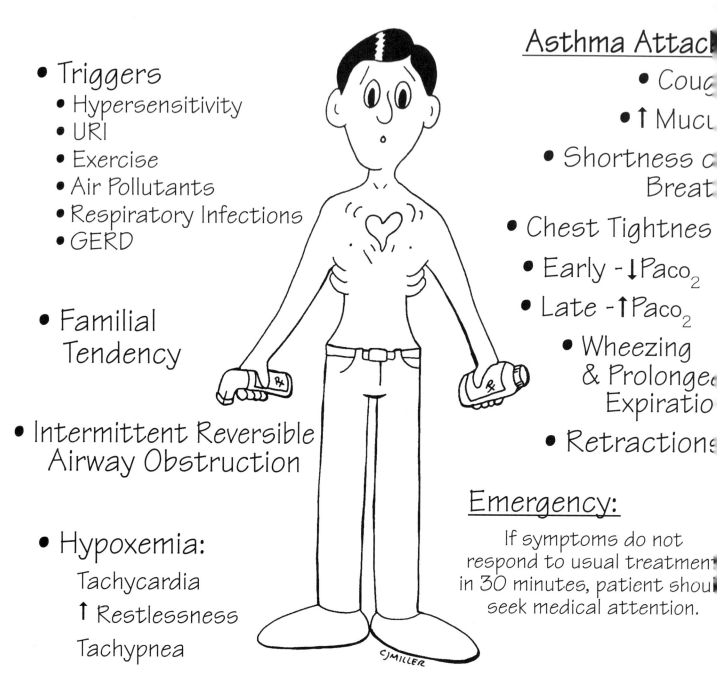

- **Triggers**
  - Hypersensitivity
  - URI
  - Exercise
  - Air Pollutants
  - Respiratory Infections
  - GERD

- **Familial Tendency**

- **Intermittent Reversible Airway Obstruction**

- **Hypoxemia:**

  Tachycardia

  ↑ Restlessness

  Tachypnea

Asthma Attac
- Coug
- ↑ Mucu
- Shortness c Breat
- Chest Tightnes
- Early - ↓$Paco_2$
- Late - ↑$Paco_2$
- Wheezing & Prolonge Expiratio
- Retractions

Emergency:

If symptoms do not respond to usual treatmen in 30 minutes, patient shou seek medical attention.

Status Asthmaticu

Can be life threatening!

Respiratory
NursingEd.com

COPD

CHRONIC AIRFLOW LIMITATION
"EMPHYSEMA AND CHRONIC BRONCHITIS"

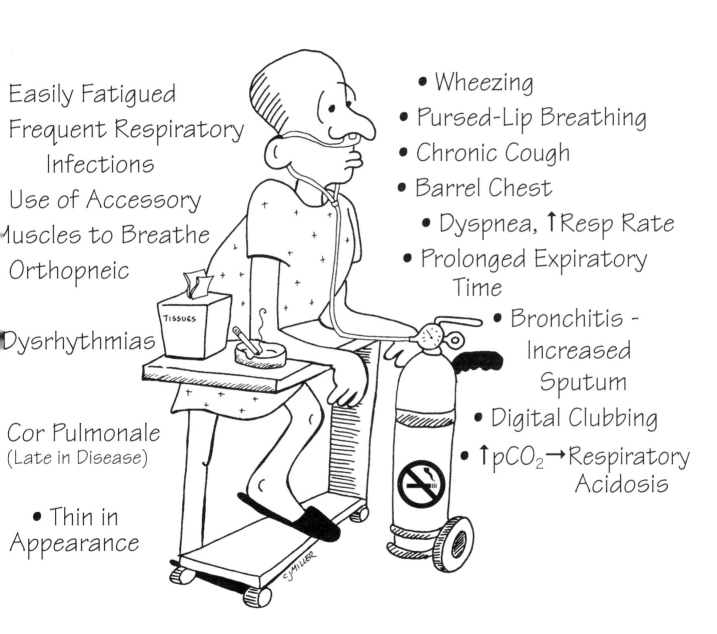

Easily Fatigued
Frequent Respiratory
Infections
Use of Accessory
Muscles to Breathe
Orthopneic

Dysrhythmias

Cor Pulmonale
(Late in Disease)

- Thin in
Appearance

- Wheezing
- Pursed-Lip Breathing
- Chronic Cough
- Barrel Chest
- Dyspnea, ↑Resp Rate
- Prolonged Expiratory
Time
- Bronchitis -
Increased
Sputum
- Digital Clubbing
- ↑pCO_2→Respiratory
Acidosis

©Nursing Education Consultants, Inc.

EMPHYSEMA
"PINK PUFFER"

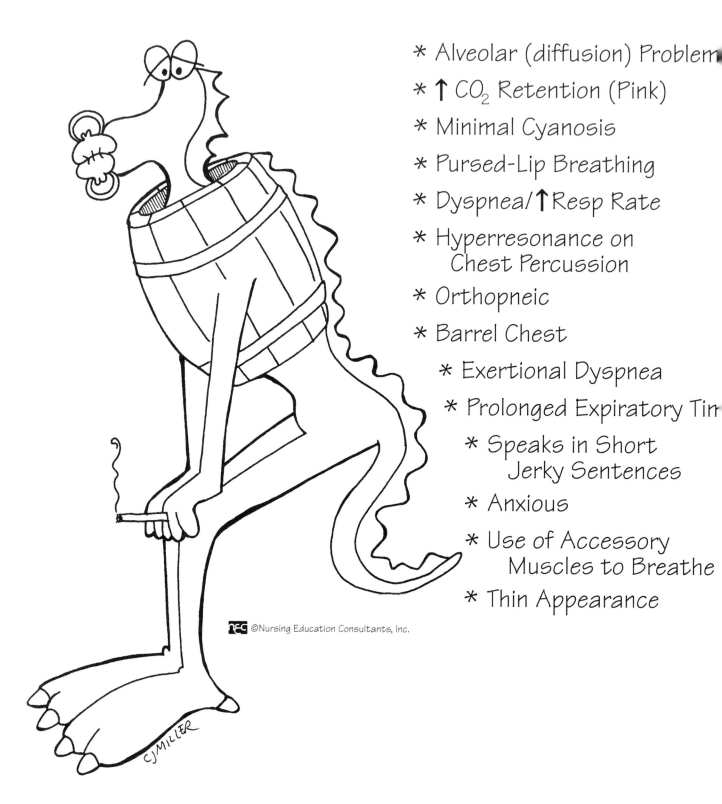

* Alveolar (diffusion) Problem
* ↑ CO_2 Retention (Pink)
* Minimal Cyanosis
* Pursed-Lip Breathing
* Dyspnea/↑ Resp Rate
* Hyperresonance on Chest Percussion
* Orthopneic
* Barrel Chest
  * Exertional Dyspnea
  * Prolonged Expiratory Time
  * Speaks in Short Jerky Sentences
  * Anxious
  * Use of Accessory Muscles to Breathe
  * Thin Appearance

©Nursing Education Consultants, Inc.

CHRONIC BRONCHITIS
"BLUE BLOATER"

Airway Flow Problem

Color Dusky to Cyanotic

Recurrent Cough &
  ↑ Sputum Production

Hypoxia

Hypercapnia (↑ pCO_2)

Respiratory Acidosis

↑ Hgb

↑ Resp Rate

Exertional Dyspnea

↑ Incidence in Smokers

Digital Clubbing

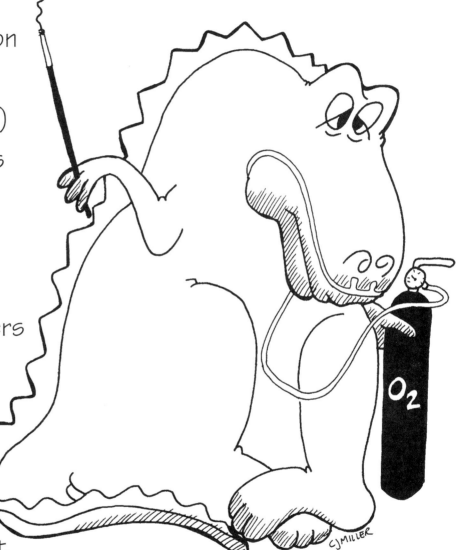

Cardiac Enlargement

Use of Accessory Muscles to Breathe

Leads to Right-Sided Heart Failure:
  Bilateral Pedal Edema, ↑ JVD

ACUTE LARYNGOTRACHEOBRONCHITIS

LTB (Croup)

- Slow Onset
- Barking Cough
- "Crowing Sounds"

- Inspiratory Stridor
- Occurs at Night in Fall and Winter
- May Progress to Hypoxic State
- May Have Slight Temperature (<102°)

- Commonly Occurs Before Age 5
- U.R.I.'s Frequently Precede LTB
- Restlessness
- Supra-sternal Retractions
- ↑Respiratory Rate

©Nursing Education Consultants, Inc.

PULMONARY EDEMA

M Meds → Nitroprusside, Morphine
A Airway
D Decrease Preload (Nitroglycerin IV)

D Diuretics (Lasix)
O Oxygen
G Blood Gases (ABG's)

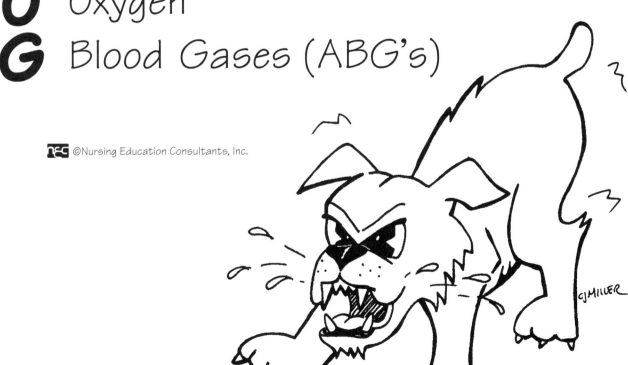

©Nursing Education Consultants, Inc.

TUBERCULOSIS (TB)

- Progressive Fatigue
- Malaise
- Anorexia
- Wt. Loss

- Chronic Cough (Productive)

- Night Sweats
- Hemoptysis (Advanced State)

- Pleuritic Chest Pai

- Low Grade Fever

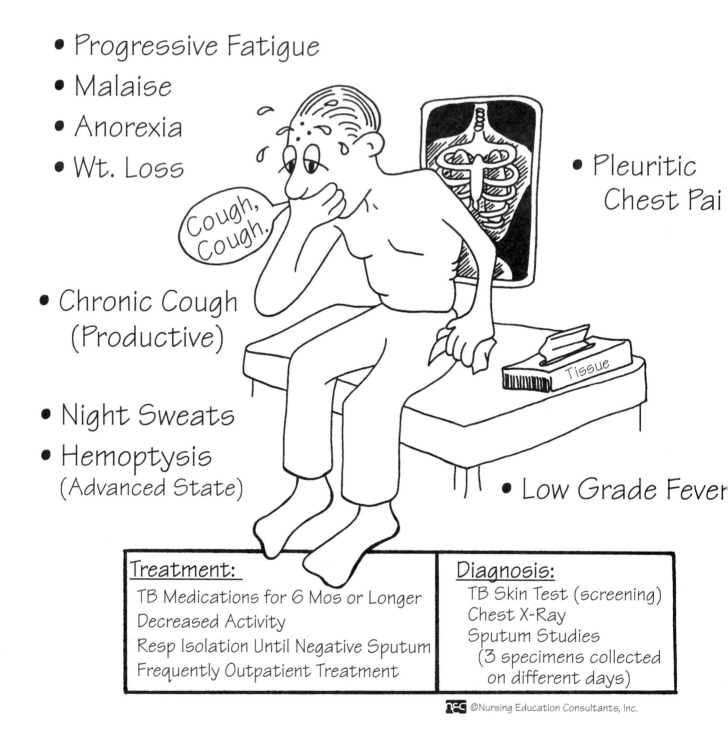

Cough, Cough,

Tissue

Treatment:
TB Medications for 6 Mos or Longer
Decreased Activity
Resp Isolation Until Negative Sputum
Frequently Outpatient Treatment

Diagnosis:
TB Skin Test (screening)
Chest X-Ray
Sputum Studies
(3 specimens collected on different days)

©Nursing Education Consultants, Inc.

SLEEP APNEA

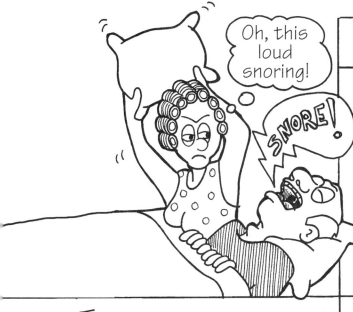

Symptoms

- Loud Snoring
- Excessive day time sleepiness
- Frequent episodes of obstructed breathing during sleep
- Morning headache
- Unrefreshing sleep
- Increased irritability

Treatments

Non-Surgical
- Change sleep position
- Decrease weight
- CPAP (Continuous Positive Airway Pressure)
- Drug Therapy for Underlying Cause

Surgical
- Adenoidectomy
- Uvulectomy
- Remodeling posterior oropharynx
- Bariatric surgery to ↓ weight

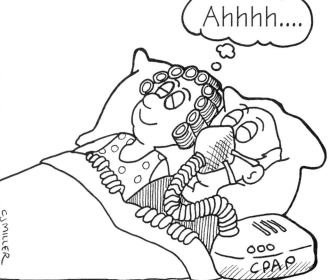

NEUROVASCULAR ASSESSMENT

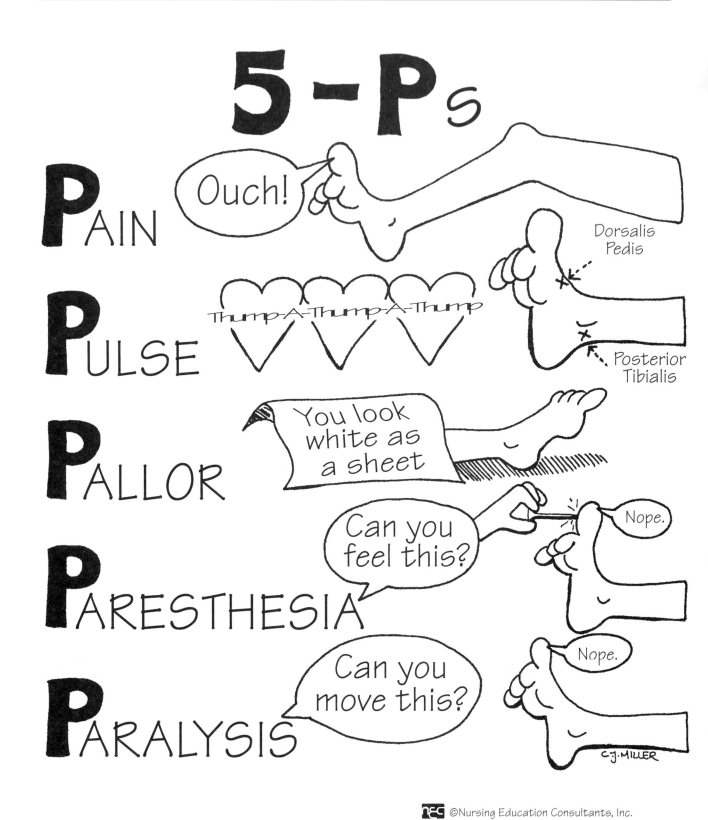

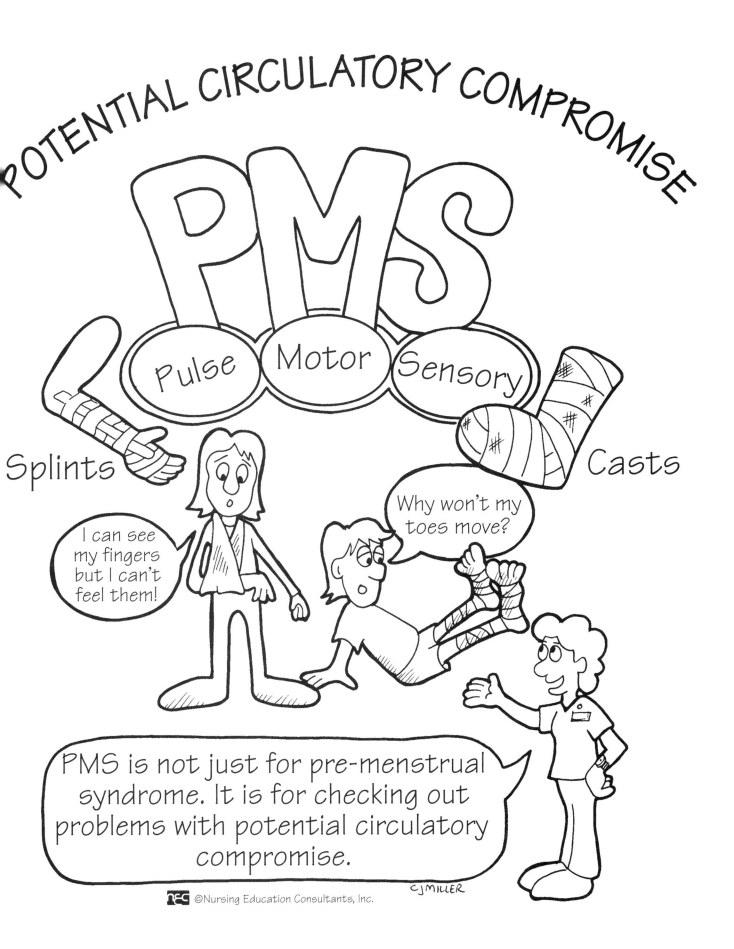

SIGNS OF SHOCK
↓ In MAP (Mean Arterial Pressure)

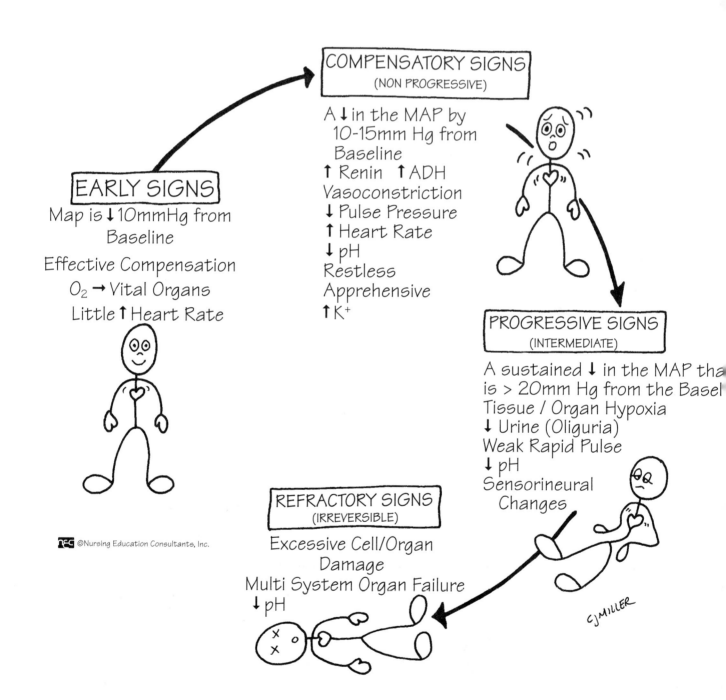

EARLY SIGNS

Map is ↓10mmHg from Baseline

Effective Compensation

O_2 → Vital Organs

Little ↑ Heart Rate

COMPENSATORY SIGNS
(NON PROGRESSIVE)

A ↓ in the MAP by 10-15mm Hg from Baseline
↑ Renin ↑ADH
Vasoconstriction
↓ Pulse Pressure
↑ Heart Rate
↓ pH
Restless
Apprehensive
↑ K^+

PROGRESSIVE SIGNS
(INTERMEDIATE)

A sustained ↓ in the MAP that is > 20mm Hg from the Basel
Tissue / Organ Hypoxia
↓ Urine (Oliguria)
Weak Rapid Pulse
↓ pH
Sensorineural Changes

REFRACTORY SIGNS
(IRREVERSIBLE)

Excessive Cell/Organ Damage
Multi System Organ Failure
↓ pH

CJMILLER

HYPERTENSION NURSING CARE

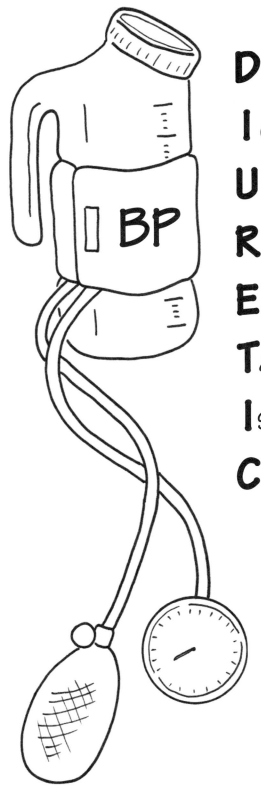

Daily weight

I & O

Urine Output

Response of B/P

Electrolytes

Take Pulses

Ischemic Episodes (TIA)

Complications: 4 C's
  CAD
  CRF
  CHF
  CVA

COMPLICATIONS OF THE TRAUMA PATIENT

T — Tissue Perfusion Problems

R — Respiratory Problems

A — Anxiety

U — Unstable Clotting Factors

M — Malnutrition (Fluids & Food)

A — Altered Body Image

T — Thromboembolism

I — Infection

C — Coping Problems

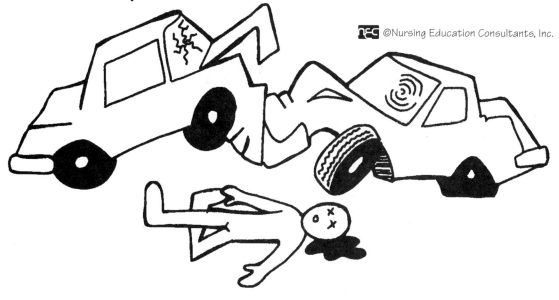

©Nursing Education Consultants, Inc.

Vascular
NursingEd.com

Aortic   Pulmonic

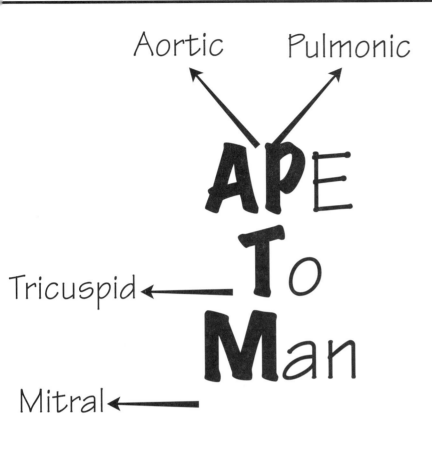

APE
   To
Tricuspid ←   **M**an

Mitral ←

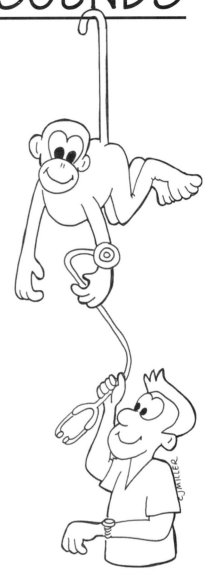

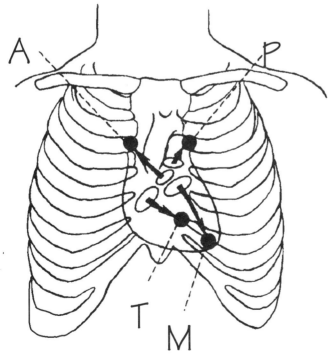

A   P

T   M

©Nursing Education Consultants, Inc.

PRELOAD AND AFTERLOAD

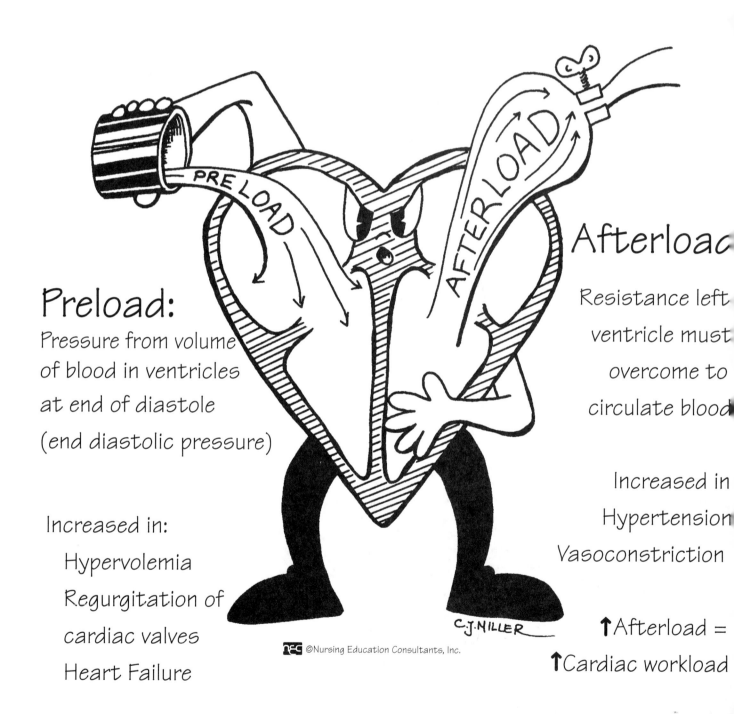

Preload:

Pressure from volume of blood in ventricles at end of diastole (end diastolic pressure)

Increased in:

Hypervolemia

Regurgitation of cardiac valves

Heart Failure

Afterload

Resistance left ventricle must overcome to circulate blood

Increased in Hypertension

Vasoconstriction

↑Afterload = ↑Cardiac workload

PEG ©Nursing Education Consultants, Inc.

C.J.MILLER

LDL/HDL

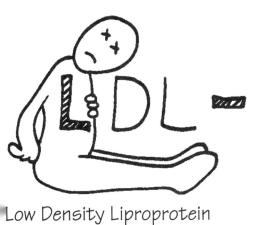

Low Density Liproprotein

Want <u>LOW</u> (↓100mg/dl) or it will lower you into the ground.

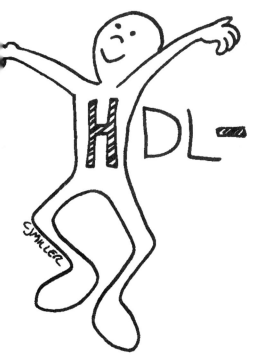

High Density Liproprotein

Want <u>HIGH</u> (↑40mg/dl) for patient to feel healthy.

©Nursing Education Consultants, Inc.

- MYOCARDIAL INFARCTION (MI) -

- CORONARY OCCLUSION -
- HEART ATTACK -

- Pain:
  - Sudden Onset
  - Substernal
  - Crushing
  - Tightness
  - Severe
  - Unrelieved by Nitro
  - May Radiate To: Back
    - Neck
    - Jaw/Tooth
    - Shoulder
    - Arm

- Dyspnea
- Syncope (↓BP)
- Nausea
- Vomiting
- Extreme Weakness
- Diaphoresis
- Denial is
  Common
- ↑Pulse
- Changes in ST
  Segment

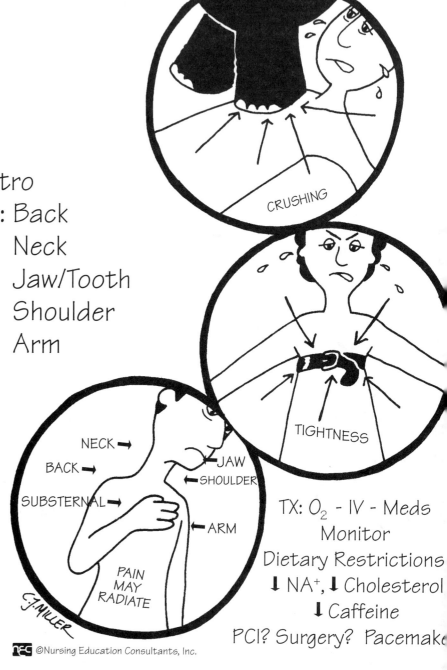

CRUSHING

TIGHTNESS

NECK →
BACK →
SUBSTERNAL →
JAW
SHOULDER
ARM
PAIN MAY RADIATE

G.MILLER

TX: O_2 - IV - Meds
Monitor
Dietary Restrictions
↓NA$^+$, ↓Cholesterol
↓Caffeine
PCI? Surgery? Pacemaker

Cardiac
NursingEd.com

LEFT SIDED ♥ FAILURE

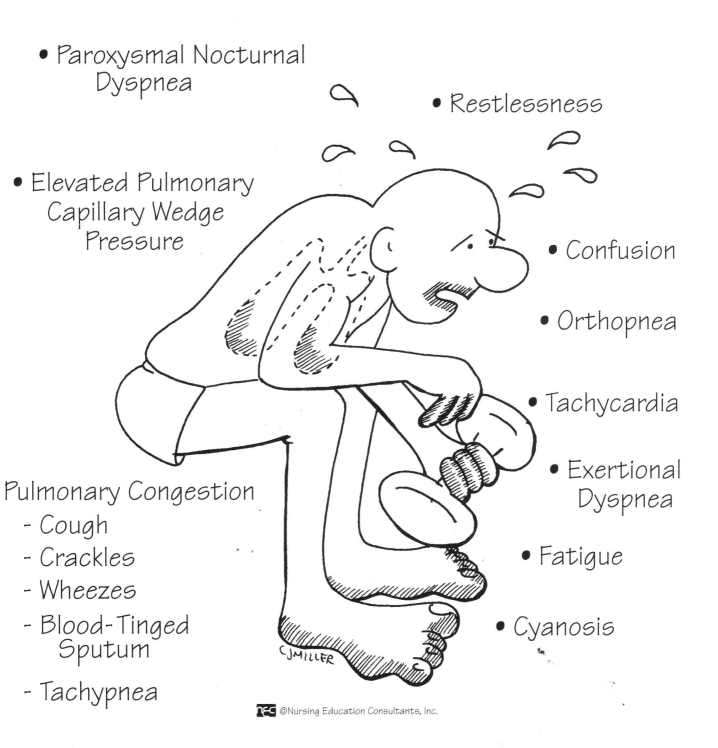

- Paroxysmal Nocturnal Dyspnea

- Elevated Pulmonary Capillary Wedge Pressure

• Restlessness

• Confusion

• Orthopnea

• Tachycardia

• Exertional Dyspnea

• Fatigue

• Cyanosis

Pulmonary Congestion
- Cough
- Crackles
- Wheezes
- Blood-Tinged Sputum
- Tachypnea

CJMILLER

RIGHT SIDED ♥ FAILURE

(Cor Pulmonale)

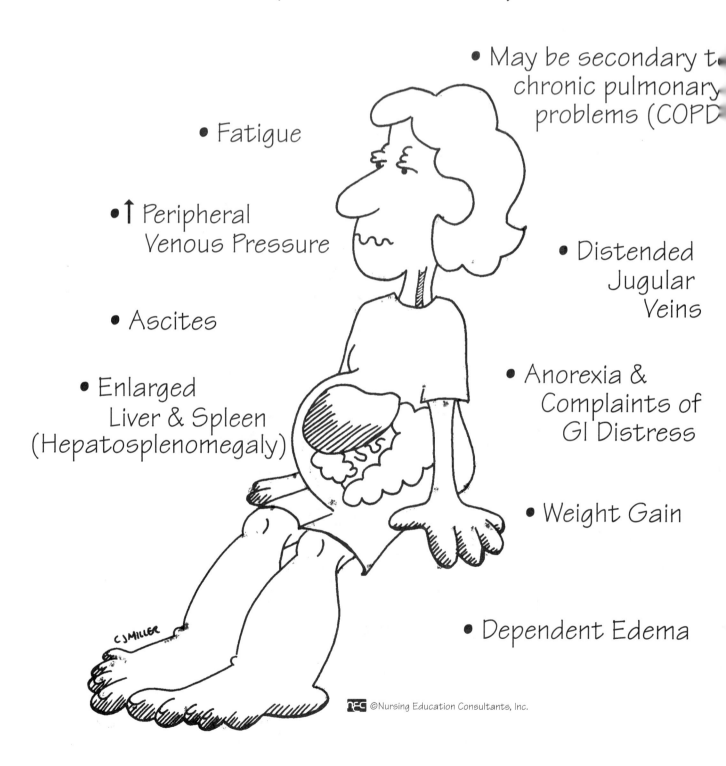

• Fatigue

• ↑ Peripheral Venous Pressure

• Ascites

• Enlarged Liver & Spleen (Hepatosplenomegaly)

• May be secondary t̶ chronic pulmonar̶ problems (COPD

• Distended Jugular Veins

• Anorexia & Complaints of GI Distress

• Weight Gain

• Dependent Edema

©Nursing Education Consultants, Inc.

Cardiac
NursingEd.com

CYANOTIC DEFECTS MNEMONIC

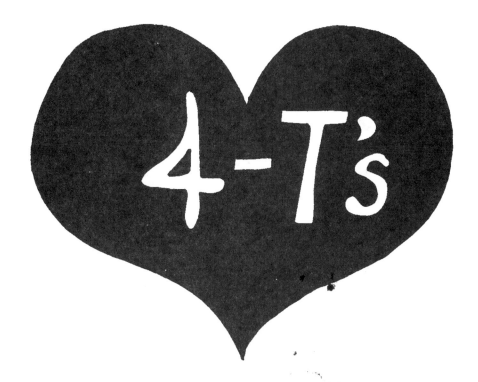

↓Pulmonary Blood Flow
- **T**etralogy of Fallot
- **T**ricuspid Atresia

Mixed Blood Flow
- **T**ransposition of Great Arteries
- **T**runcus Arteriosus

CONGENITAL ❤ DEFECTS

↓Pulmonary Blood Flow

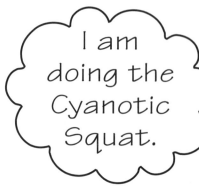

Example:
Tetralogy of Fallot
Tricuspid Atresia

- Squatting
- Cyanosis
- Clubbing
- Syncope

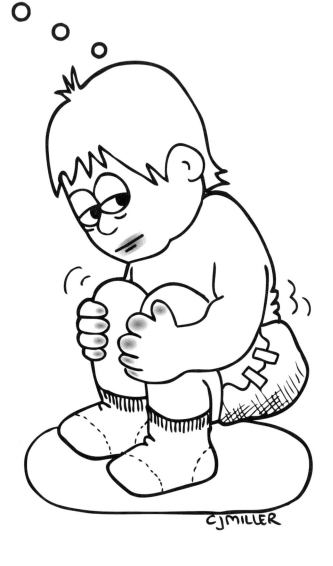

CJMILLER

Cardiac
NursingEd.com

CONGENITAL 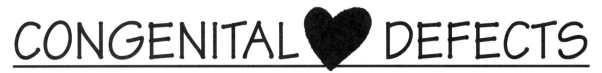 DEFECTS

↑Pulmonary Blood Flow

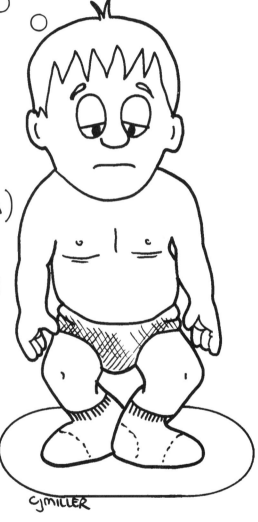

I'm not blue, just tired all the time.

Example:
Patent Ductus Arteriosus (PDA)
Atrial Septal Defect (ASD)
Ventricular Septal Defect (VSD)

↑ Fatigue
♡ Murmur
↑ Risk Endocarditis
CHF
Growth Retardation

CJMILLER

CONGENITAL ♥ DEFECT
SYMPTOMS

- ♥ ↑ Pulse
- ♥ ↑ Respirations
- ♥ Retarded Growth
- ♥ Dyspnea, Orthopnea
- ♥ Fatigue
- ♥ URI

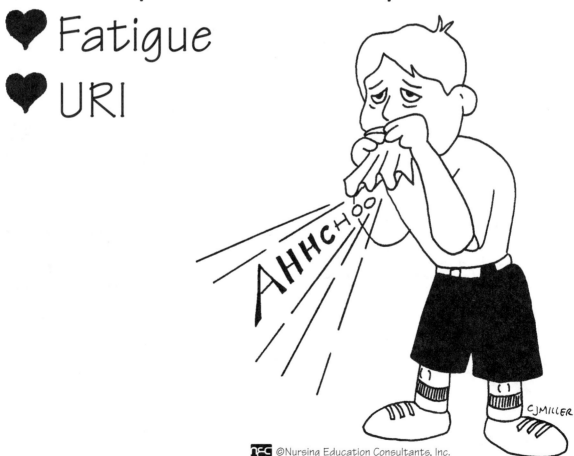

AHHCHOO

CJMILLER

Cardiac
NursingEd.com

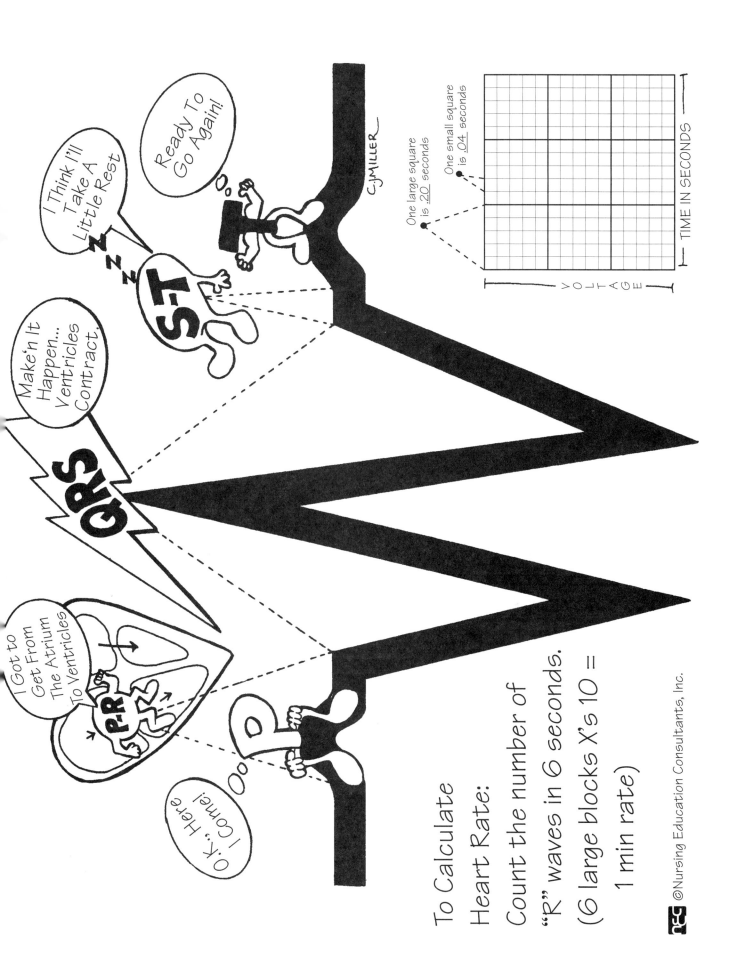

CARDIAC
ELECTROPHYSIOLOGY

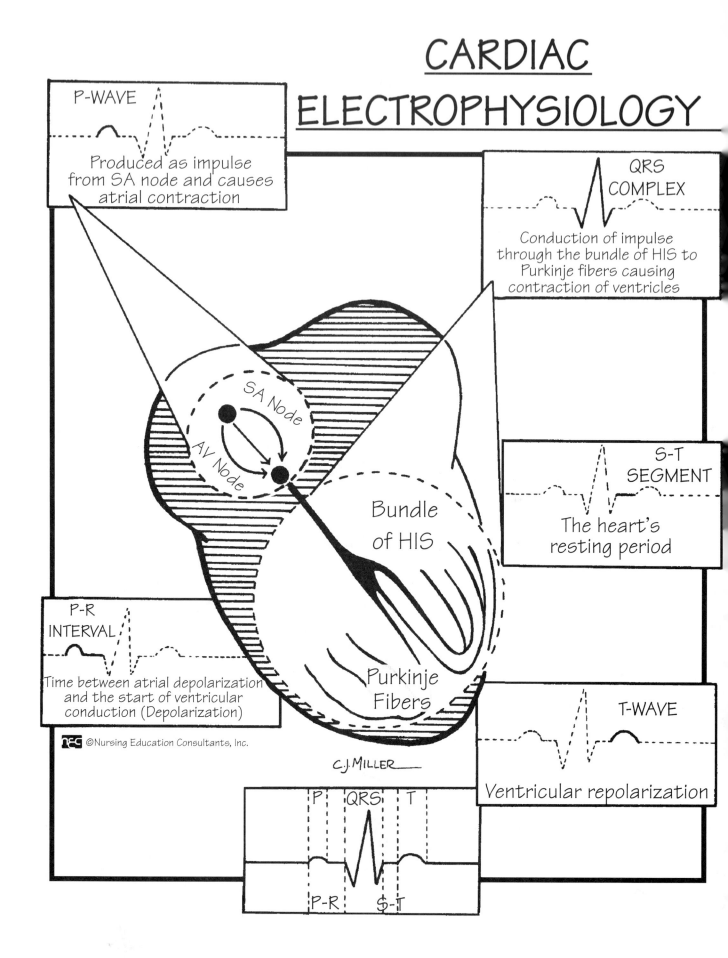

P-WAVE

Produced as impulse from SA node and causes atrial contraction

QRS COMPLEX

Conduction of impulse through the bundle of HIS to Purkinje fibers causing contraction of ventricles

S-T SEGMENT

The heart's resting period

P-R INTERVAL

Time between atrial depolarization and the start of ventricular conduction (Depolarization)

T-WAVE

Ventricular repolarization

SA Node

AV Node

Bundle of HIS

Purkinje Fibers

P QRS T

P-R S-T

©Nursing Education Consultants, Inc.

C.J. MILLER

88

Cardiac
NursingEd.com

© 2012 Nursing Education
Consultants, Inc.

PEPTIC ULCER DISEASE (PUD)

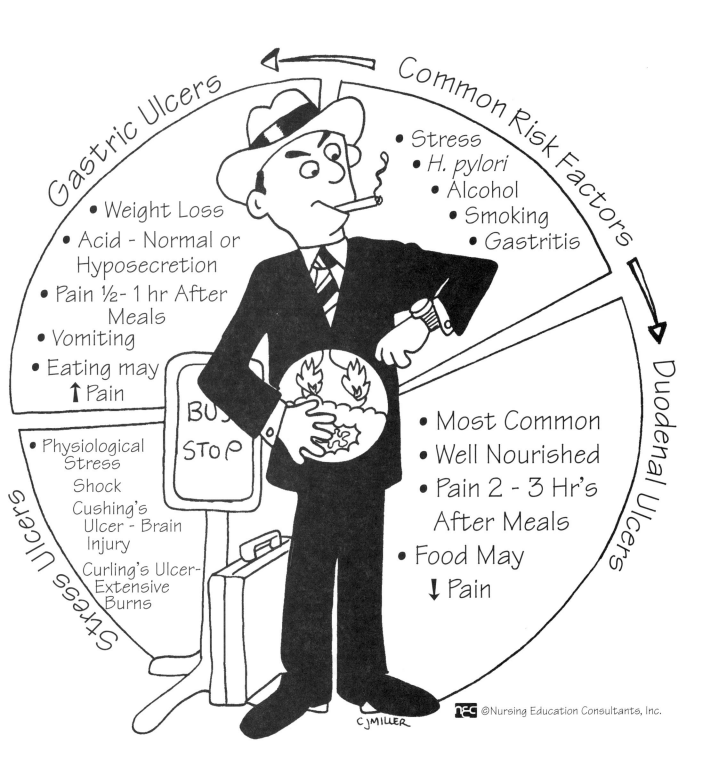

Gastric Ulcers
- Weight Loss
- Acid - Normal or Hyposecretion
- Pain ½ - 1 hr After Meals
- Vomiting
- Eating may ↑ Pain

Common Risk Factors
- Stress
- *H. pylori*
- Alcohol
- Smoking
- Gastritis

Stress Ulcers
- Physiological Stress
  Shock
  Cushing's Ulcer - Brain Injury
  Curling's Ulcer - Extensive Burns

Duodenal Ulcers
- Most Common
- Well Nourished
- Pain 2 - 3 Hr's After Meals
- Food May ↓ Pain

BUS STOP

CJMILLER   ©Nursing Education Consultants, Inc.

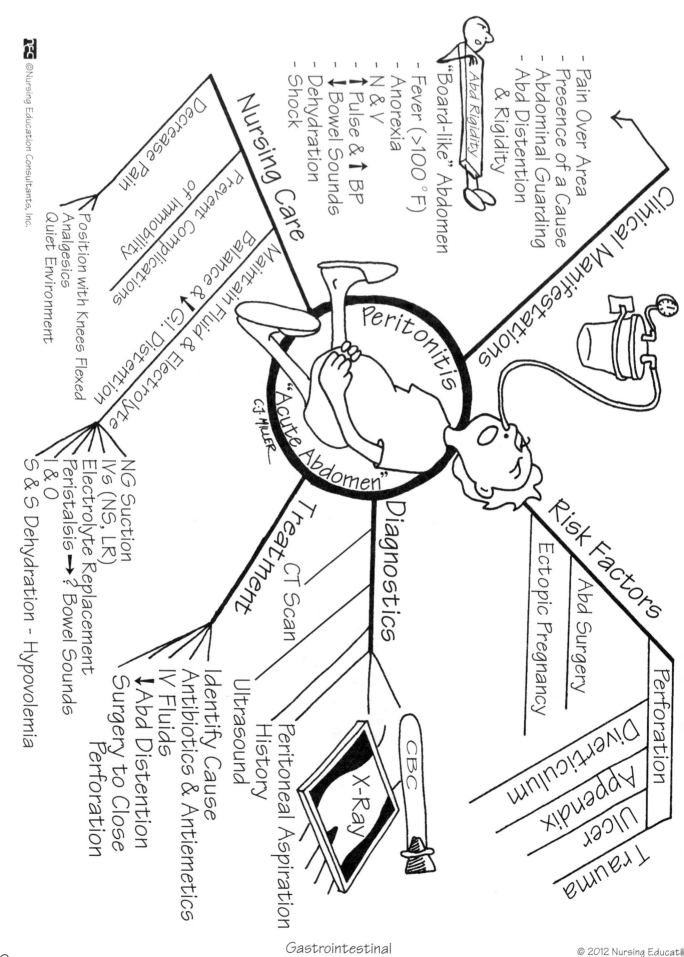

Peritonitis

"Acute Abdomen"

C.J. Miller

Clinical Manifestations

Abd Rigidity

- Pain Over Area
- Presence of a Cause
- Abdominal Guarding
- Abd Distention & Rigidity
- "Board-like" Abdomen
- Fever (>100 °F)
- Anorexia
- N & V
- ↑ Pulse & ↑ BP
- ↕ Bowel Sounds
- Dehydration
- Shock

Nursing Care

Decrease Pain
- Position with Knees Flexed
- Analgesics
- Quiet Environment

Prevent Complications of Immobility

Balance & ↓ G.I. Distention

Maintain Fluid & Electrolyte
- NG Suction
- IVs (NS, LR)
- Electrolyte Replacement
- Peristalsis → ↓ Bowel Sounds
- I & O
- S & S Dehydration - Hypovolemia

Treatment

- Identify Cause
- Antibiotics & Antiemetics
- IV Fluids
- ↓ Abd Distention
- Surgery to Close Perforation

Diagnostics

- CT Scan
- Ultrasound
- History
- Peritoneal Aspiration
- X-Ray
- CBC

Risk Factors

- Ectopic Pregnancy
- Abd Surgery
- Perforation
- Diverticulum
- Appendix
- Ulcer
- Trauma

CROHN'S DISEASE

Occurs Teens to Mid-30s

Second Peak After
　Age 60

? Autoimmune
　Factors

Nausea & Vomiting

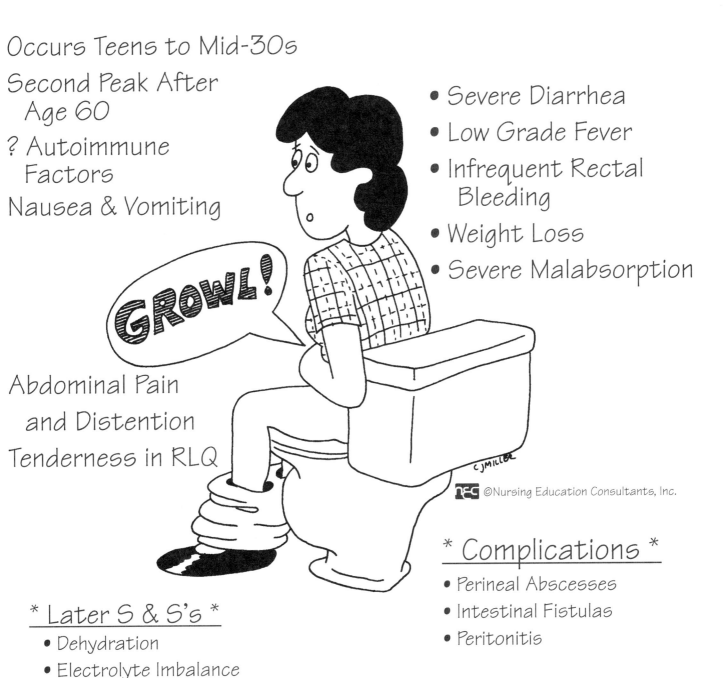

GROWL!

- Severe Diarrhea
- Low Grade Fever
- Infrequent Rectal
　Bleeding
- Weight Loss
- Severe Malabsorption

Abdominal Pain
　and Distention

Tenderness in RLQ

©Nursing Education Consultants, Inc.

* Later S & S's *
- Dehydration
- Electrolyte Imbalance
- Anemia

* Complications *
- Perineal Abscesses
- Intestinal Fistulas
- Peritonitis

HEPATIC ENCEPHALOPATHY

HEPATIC COMA

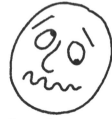

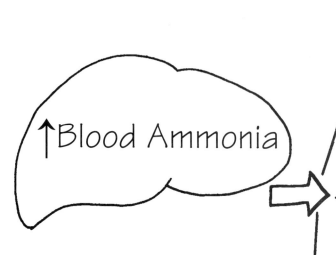

↑Blood Ammonia

⊙ Changes in LOC
- Progressive Confusion
- Stuporous
- Impaired Thinking & Judgment

⊙ Neuromuscular Disturbances
- Asterixis
  "Liver Flap"
- Hyperreflexia
- Fetor Hepaticus

Problem ↑'d By:

- Constipation
- Infection
- Hypovolemia
- Hypokalemia (↓K)
- GI Bleeding
- Opioid Meds

⊙ Treatment

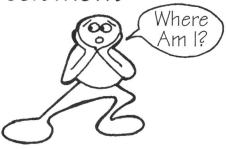

- Administer Vancomycin & Lactulose
- Administer Cathartics & Enemas
- Promote Diet ↑ in Carbohydrates & Adequate Fluids

Liver
NursingEd.com

CIRRHOSIS:
LATER CLINICAL MANIFESTATIONS

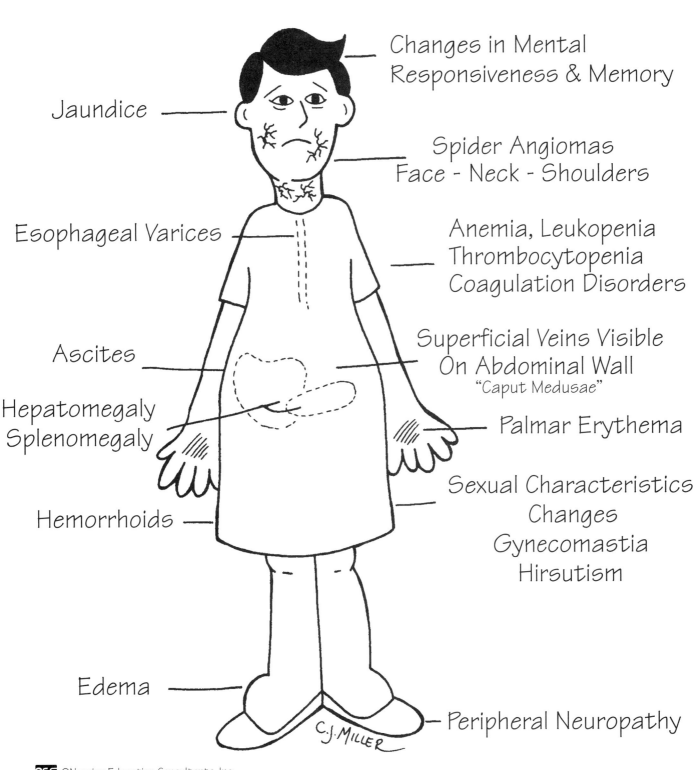

Changes in Mental
Responsiveness & Memory

Jaundice

Spider Angiomas
Face - Neck - Shoulders

Esophageal Varices

Anemia, Leukopenia
Thrombocytopenia
Coagulation Disorders

Ascites

Superficial Veins Visible
On Abdominal Wall
"Caput Medusae"

Hepatomegaly
Splenomegaly

Palmar Erythema

Hemorrhoids

Sexual Characteristics
Changes
Gynecomastia
Hirsutism

Edema

Peripheral Neuropathy

C.J. MILLER

2012 Nursing Education
nsultants, Inc.

CHOLECYSTITIS

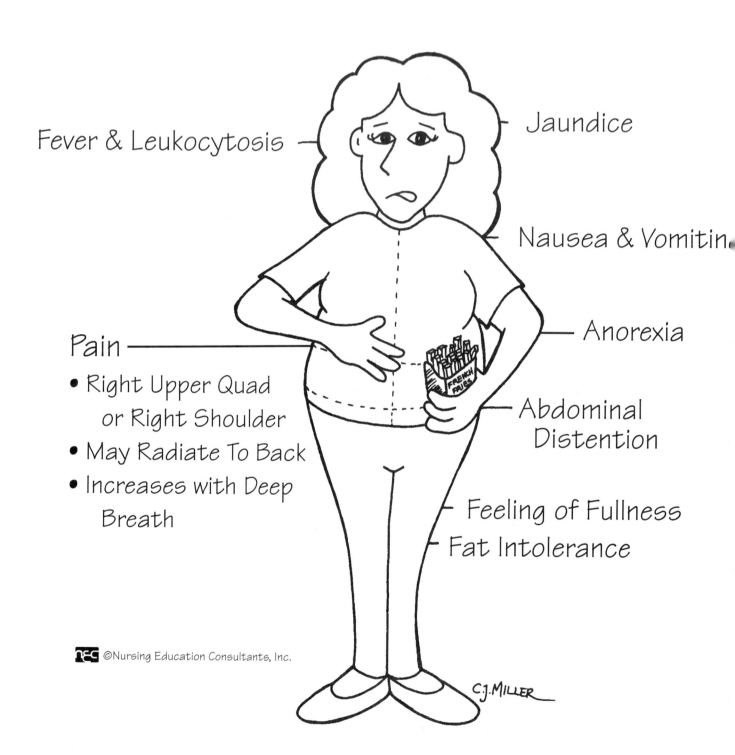

Fever & Leukocytosis

Jaundice

Nausea & Vomitin...

Anorexia

Pain
- Right Upper Quad or Right Shoulder
- May Radiate To Back
- Increases with Deep Breath

Abdominal Distention

Feeling of Fullness

Fat Intolerance

C.J.MILLER

Liver
NursingEd.com

HEPATITIS A & E

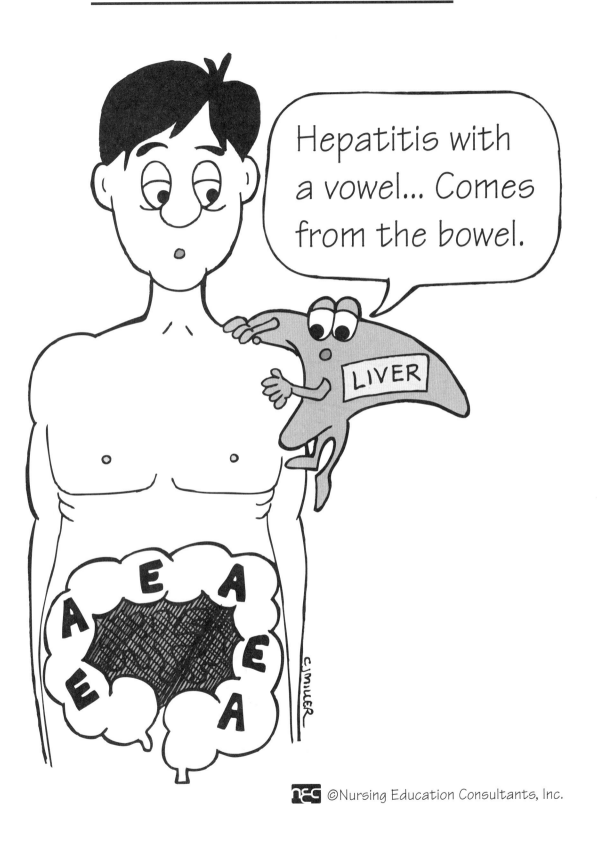

ABNORMAL POSTURING

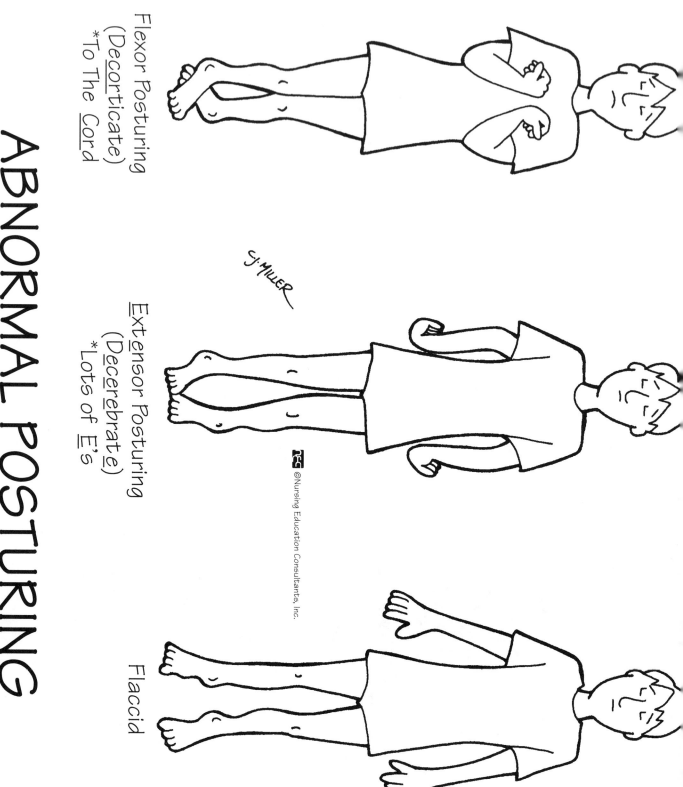

Flexor Posturing
(De̲cortic̲ate)
*To The C̲ord

Ex̲tensor Posturing
(De̲cer̲ebrat̲e)
*Lots of E̲'s

Flaccid

S.J. Miller

©Nursing Education Consultants, Inc.

CRANIAL NERVE MNEMONIC

S = Sensory	M = Motor	B = Both

O	Olfactory	O	On	S	Some
O	Optic	O	Old	S	Say
O	Oculomotor	O	Olympus	M	Marry
T	Trochlear	T	Towering	M	Money
T	Trigeminal	T	Tops	B	But
A	Abducens	A	A	M	My
F	Facial	F	Finn	B	Brother
A	Acoustic	A	And	S	Says
G	Glossopharyngeal	G	German	B	Bad
V	Vagus Nerve	V	Viewed	B	Business
S	Spinal	S	Some	M	Marry
H	Hypoglossal	H	Hops	M	Money

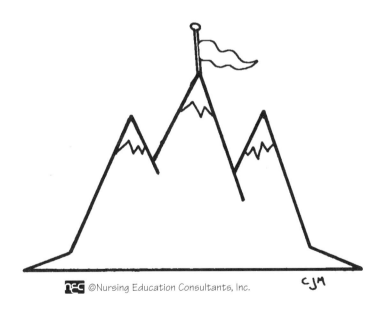

nec ©Nursing Education Consultants, Inc.

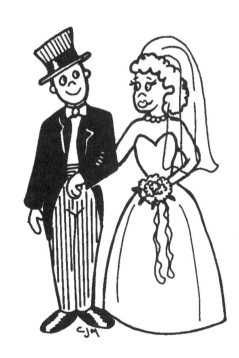

INCREASED INTRACRANIAL PRESSURE

- Changes in LOC
  - Flattening of Affect
  - ↓ Orientation & Attention
  - Coma

- Eyes
  - Papilledema
  - Pupillary Changes
  - Impaired
    Eye Movement

- Posturing
  - Decerebrate
  - Decorticate
  - Flaccid

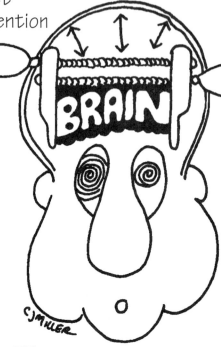

©Nursing Education Consultants, Inc.

- Decreased
  Motor Function
  - Change in Motor Ability
  - Posturing

- Headache

- Seizures
  - Impaired Sensory
    & Motor Function

- Changes in
  Vital Signs:
  - Cushing's Triad:
    - ↑ Systolic BP
      "Widening Pulse Pressure"
    - ↓ Pulse
    - Irregular
      Resp Pattern

- Vomiting
  - Not Preceded by Nause
  - May be Projectile

- Changes in Speech

◎ Infants: ○ Bulging Fontanels
○ Cranial Suture Separation
○ ↑ Head Circumference
○ High Pitched Cry

Neurology
NursingEd.com

INCREASED INTRACRANIAL PRESSURE (IICP) - CUSHING'S TRIAD

(Symptoms Of IICP Are Opposite Of Shock)

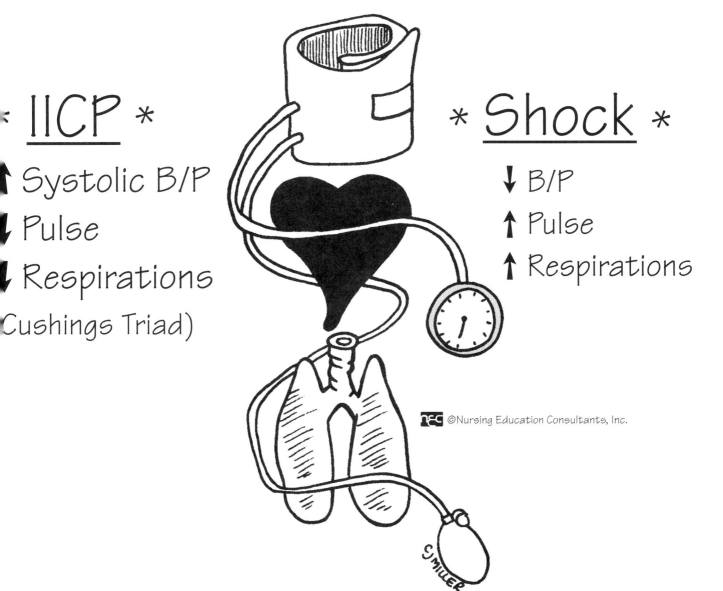

IICP *

↑ Systolic B/P

↓ Pulse

↓ Respirations

(Cushings Triad)

* Shock *

↓ B/P

↑ Pulse

↑ Respirations

©Nursing Education Consultants, Inc.

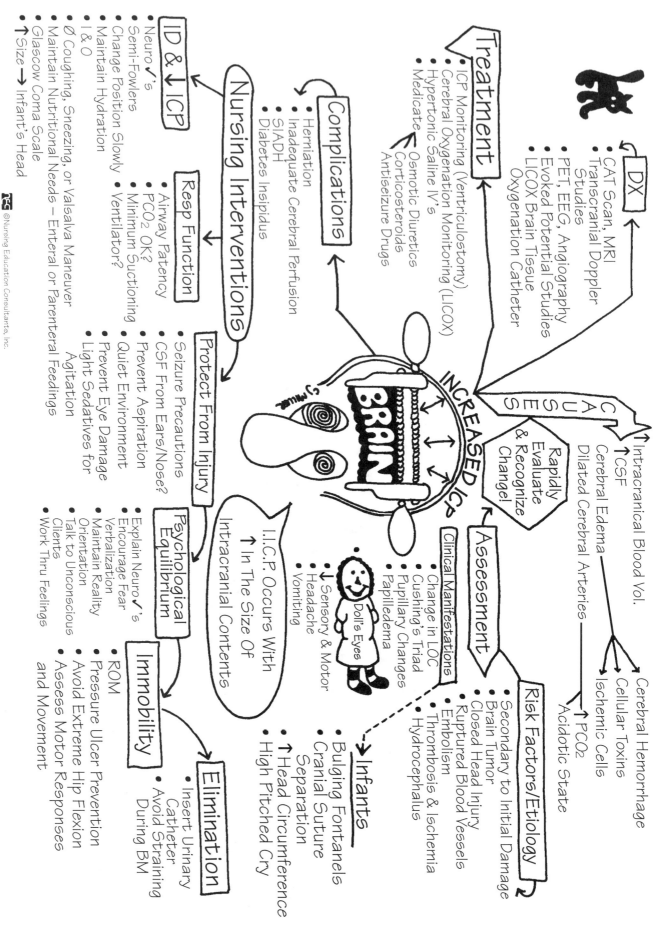

INCREASED ICP

BRAIN

Treatment
- ICP Monitoring (Ventriculostomy)
- Cerebral Oxygenation Monitoring (LICOX)
- Hypertonic Saline IV's
- Medicate
  - Osmotic Diuretics
  - Corticosteroids
  - Antiseizure Drugs

DX
- CAT Scan, MRI
- Transcranial Doppler Studies
- PET, EEG, Angiography
- Evoked Potential Studies
- LICOX Brain Tissue Oxygenation Catheter

Complications
- Herniation
- Inadequate Cerebral Perfusion
- SIADH
- Diabetes Insipidus

Nursing Interventions

ID & ↓ICP
- Neuro ✓'s
- Semi-Fowlers
- Change Position Slowly
- Maintain Hydration
- I & O
- Ø Coughing, Sneezing, or Valsalva Maneuver
- Maintain Nutritional Needs – Enteral or Parenteral Feedings
- Glascow Coma Scale
- → Size → Infant's Head

Resp Function
- Airway Patency
- PCO₂ OK?
- Minimum Suctioning
- Ventilator?

Protect From Injury
- Seizure Precautions
- CSF From Ears/Nose?
- Prevent Aspiration
- Quiet Environment
- Prevent Eye Damage
- Light Sedatives for Agitation

Psychological Equilibrium
- Explain Neuro ✓'s
- Encourage Fear Verbalization
- Maintain Reality Orientation
- Talk to Unconscious Clients
- Work Thru Feelings

I.I.C.P. Occurs With ↑ In The Size Of Intracranial Contents

Immobility
- ROM
- Pressure Ulcer Prevention
- Avoid Extreme Hip Flexion
- Assess Motor Responses and Movement

Elimination
- Insert Urinary Catheter
- Avoid Straining During BM

Clinical Manifestations
- Change in LOC
- Cushing's Triad
- Pupillary Changes
- Papilledema
- Sensory & Motor
- Headache
- Vomiting

Doll's Eyes

Infants
- Bulging Fontanels
- Cranial Suture Separation
- ↑ Head Circumference
- High Pitched Cry

Assessment

Rapidly Evaluate & Recognize Change!

C A U S E S

Risk Factors/Etiology
- Secondary to Initial Damage
- Brain Tumor
- Closed Head Injury
- Ruptured Blood Vessels
- Embolism
- Thrombosis & Ischemia
- Hydrocephalus

- ↑CSF
- ↑ Intracranical Blood Vol.
- Cerebral Edema
- Dilated Cerebral Arteries —
  - Cerebral Hemorrhage
  - Cellular Toxins
  - Ischemic Cells
  - Acidotic State
  - ↑ PCO₂

Neurology
NursingEd.com

STROKE
BRAIN ATTACK, CVA

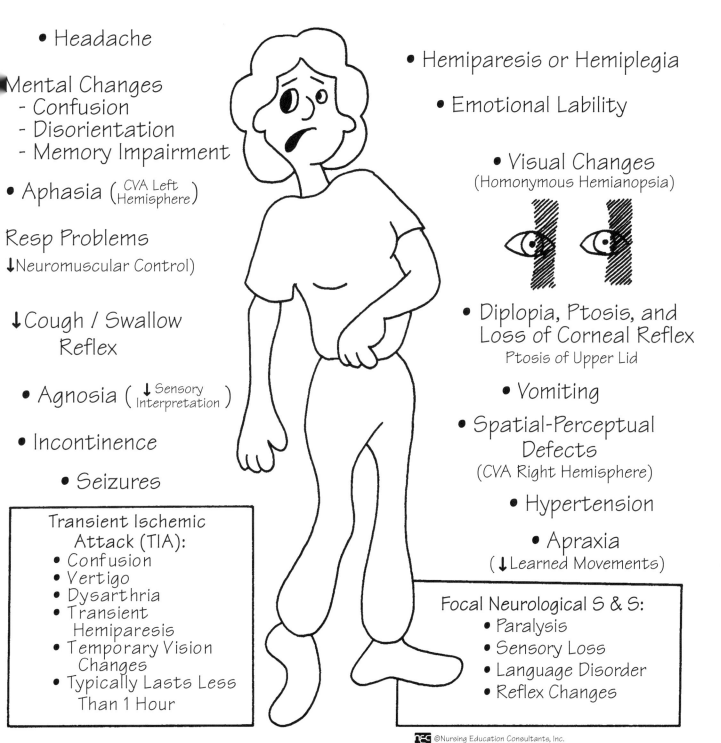

- Headache

Mental Changes
- Confusion
- Disorientation
- Memory Impairment

- Aphasia (CVA Left Hemisphere)

Resp Problems
↓Neuromuscular Control)

↓Cough / Swallow Reflex

- Agnosia (↓Sensory Interpretation)

- Incontinence

- Seizures

Transient Ischemic Attack (TIA):
- Confusion
- Vertigo
- Dysarthria
- Transient Hemiparesis
- Temporary Vision Changes
- Typically Lasts Less Than 1 Hour

- Hemiparesis or Hemiplegia

- Emotional Lability

- Visual Changes
(Homonymous Hemianopsia)

- Diplopia, Ptosis, and Loss of Corneal Reflex
Ptosis of Upper Lid

- Vomiting

- Spatial-Perceptual Defects
(CVA Right Hemisphere)

- Hypertension

- Apraxia
(↓Learned Movements)

Focal Neurological S & S:
- Paralysis
- Sensory Loss
- Language Disorder
- Reflex Changes

Stroke (Brain Accident, CVA)

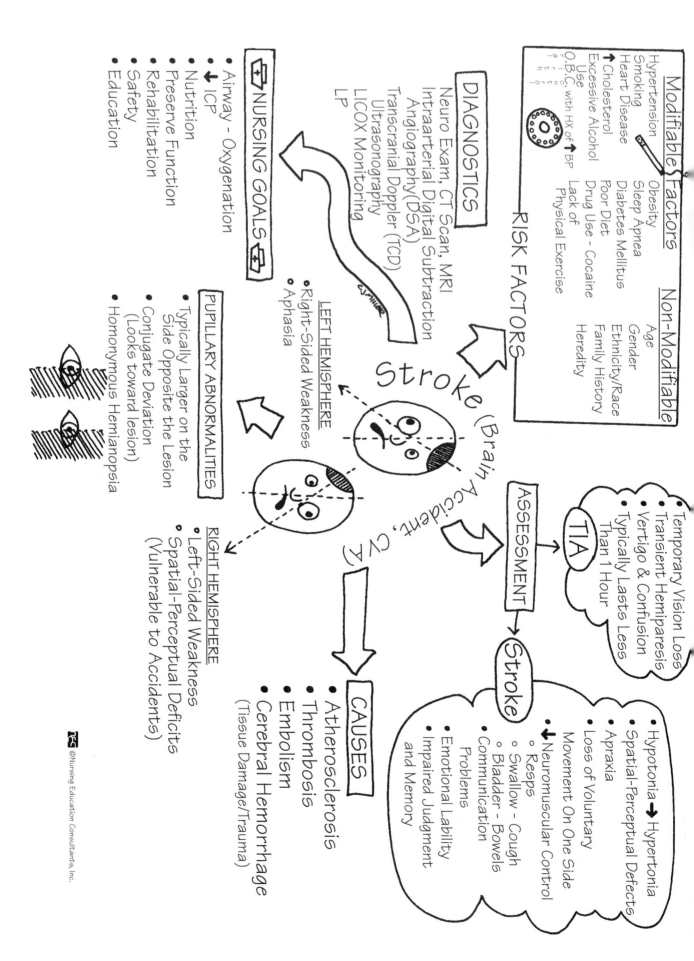

Modifiable Factors
- Hypertension
- Smoking
- → Heart Disease
- → Cholesterol
- Excessive Alcohol Use
- O.B.C. with HX of → BP
- Obesity
- Sleep Apnea
- Diabetes Mellitus
- Poor Diet
- Drug Use - Cocaine
- Lack of Physical Exercise

Non-Modifiable
- Age
- Gender
- Ethnicity/Race
- Family History
- Heredity

RISK FACTORS

DIAGNOSTICS
- Neuro Exam, CT Scan, MRI
- Intraarterial Digital Subtraction Angiography (DSA)
- Transcranial Doppler (TCD)
- Ultrasonography
- LICOX Monitoring
- LP

NURSING GOALS
- Airway - Oxygenation
- ← ICP
- Nutrition
- Preserve Function
- Rehabilitation
- Safety
- Education

LEFT HEMISPHERE
- Right-Sided Weakness
- Aphasia

RIGHT HEMISPHERE
- Left-Sided Weakness
- Spatial-Perceptual Deficits (Vulnerable to Accidents)

PUPILLARY ABNORMALITIES
- Typically Larger on the Side Opposite the Lesion
- Conjugate Deviation (Looks toward lesion)
- Homonymous Hemianopsia

ASSESSMENT

TIA
- Temporary Vision Loss
- Transient Hemiparesis
- Vertigo & Confusion
- Typically Lasts Less Than 1 Hour

Stroke
- Hypotonia → Hypertonia
- Spatial-Perceptual Defects
- Apraxia
- Loss of Voluntary Movement On One Side
- → Neuromuscular Control
  - Resps
  - Swallow - Cough
  - Bladder - Bowels
- Communication Problems
- Emotional Lability
- Impaired Judgment and Memory

CAUSES
- Atherosclerosis
- Thrombosis
- Embolism
- Cerebral Hemorrhage (Tissue Damage/Trauma)

FAST RECOGNITION OF A STROKE

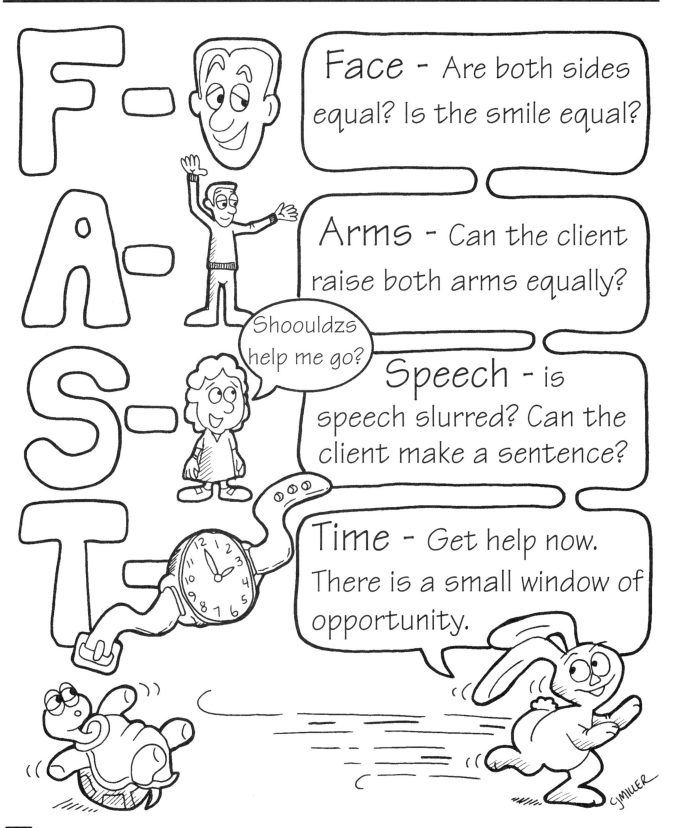

Face - Are both sides equal? Is the smile equal?

Arms - Can the client raise both arms equally?

Shoouldzs help me go?

Speech - is speech slurred? Can the client make a sentence?

Time - Get help now. There is a small window of opportunity.

PARKINSON'S DISEASE

- Onset usually gradual, after age 50. (Slowly progressive)

- Mask-Like, Blank Expression

- Stooped Posture

- Pill Rolling Tremors

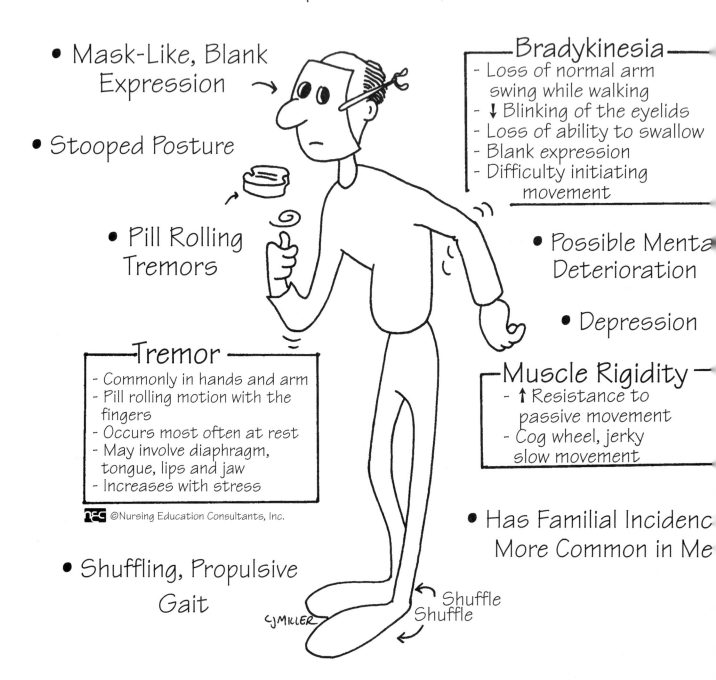

Bradykinesia
- Loss of normal arm swing while walking
- ↓ Blinking of the eyelids
- Loss of ability to swallow
- Blank expression
- Difficulty initiating movement

- Possible Mental Deterioration

- Depression

Tremor
- Commonly in hands and arm
- Pill rolling motion with the fingers
- Occurs most often at rest
- May involve diaphragm, tongue, lips and jaw
- Increases with stress

©Nursing Education Consultants, Inc.

Muscle Rigidity
- ↑ Resistance to passive movement
- Cog wheel, jerky slow movement

- Has Familial Incidence More Common in Me

- Shuffling, Propulsive Gait

CJMILLER

Shuffle Shuffle

BELL'S PALSY

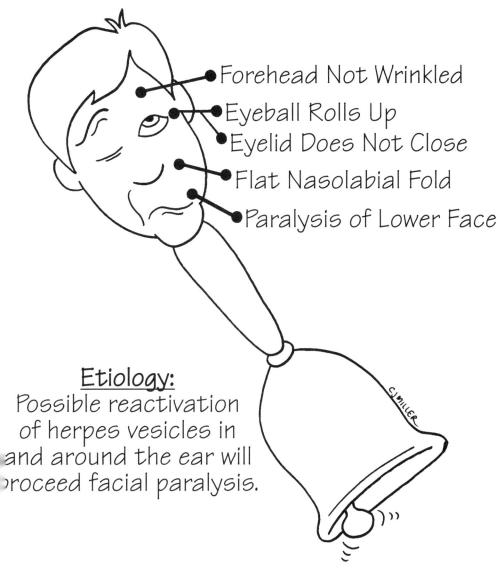

Forehead Not Wrinkled

Eyeball Rolls Up

Eyelid Does Not Close

Flat Nasolabial Fold

Paralysis of Lower Face

Etiology:
Possible reactivation of herpes vesicles in and around the ear will proceed facial paralysis.

©Nursing Education Consultants, Inc.

Treatment:
- Corticosteroids
- Antivirals
- Full Recovery in Most Patients in 6 Months, Especially if Treatment is Started Immediately

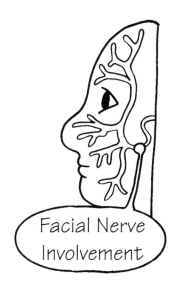

Facial Nerve Involvement

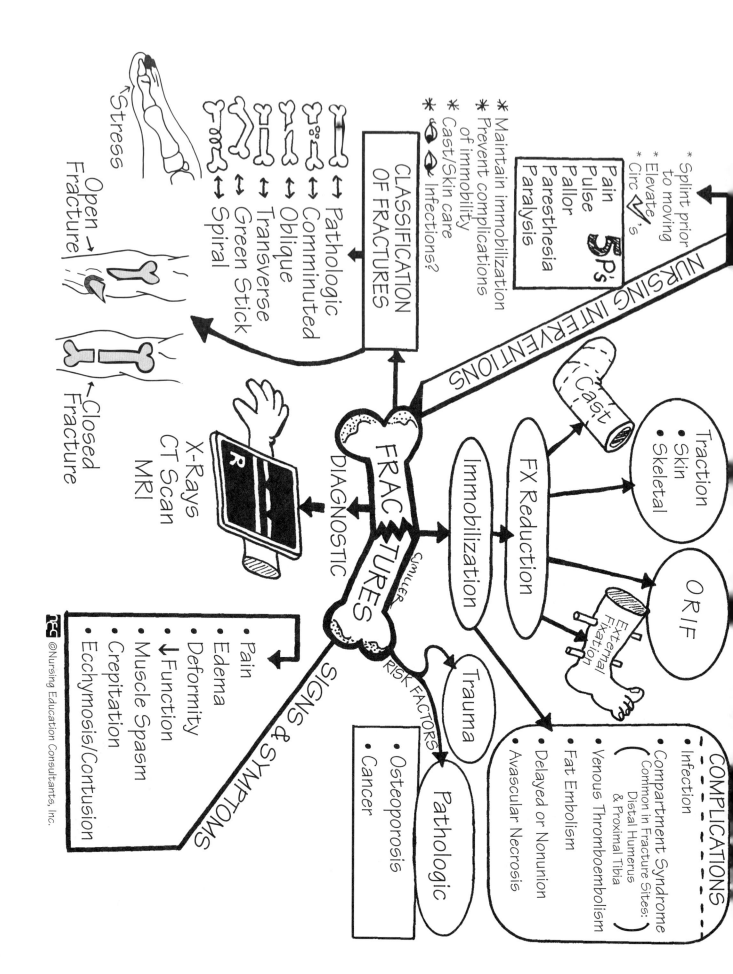

FRACTURES

C. Miller

CLASSIFICATION OF FRACTURES

- Pathologic
- Comminuted
- Oblique
- Transverse
- Green Stick
- Spiral

↑Stress
Fracture

Open Fracture →

←Closed Fracture

NURSING INTERVENTIONS

* Splint prior to moving
* Elevate
* Circ V's

5 P's:
Pain
Pulse
Pallor
Paresthesia
Paralysis

* Maintain immobilization
* Prevent complications of immobility
* Cast/Skin care
* Infections?

DIAGNOSTIC

- X-Rays
- CT Scan
- MRI

SIGNS & SYMPTOMS

- Pain
- Edema
- Deformity
- ↓Function
- Muscle Spasm
- Crepitation
- Ecchymosis/Contusion

Immobilization

FX Reduction

- Cast
- Traction
  - Skin
  - Skeletal
- ORIF
- External Fixation

RISK FACTORS

Trauma

Pathologic
- Osteoporosis
- Cancer

COMPLICATIONS

- Infection
- Compartment Syndrome (Common in Fracture Sites: Distal Humerus & Proximal Tibia)
- Venous Thromboembolism
- Fat Embolism
- Delayed or Nonunion
- Avascular Necrosis

Musculoskeletal
NursingEd.com

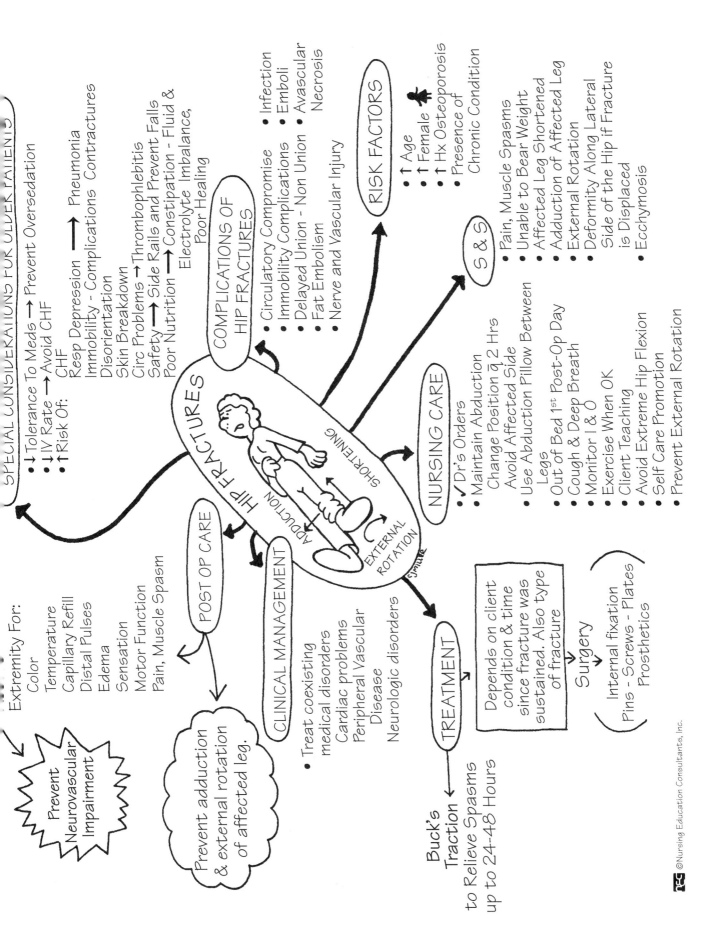

HIP FRACTURES

SPECIAL CONSIDERATIONS FOR OLDER PATIENT

- ↓Tolerance To Meds → Prevent Oversedation
- ↓IV Rate → Avoid CHF
- ↑Risk Of:
  - CHF
  - Resp Depression → Pneumonia
  - Immobility - Complications - Contractures
  - Disorientation
  - Skin Breakdown
  - Circ Problems → Thrombophlebitis
  - Safety → Side Rails and Prevent Falls
  - Poor Nutrition → Constipation - Fluid & Electrolyte Imbalance, Poor Healing

COMPLICATIONS OF HIP FRACTURES

- Circulatory Compromise
- Immobility Complications
- Delayed Union - Non Union
- Fat Embolism
- Nerve and Vascular Injury
- Infection
- Emboli
- Avascular Necrosis

RISK FACTORS

- ↑ Age
- ↑ Female
- ↑ Hx Osteoporosis
- Presence of Chronic Condition

S & S

- Pain, Muscle Spasms
- Unable to Bear Weight
- Affected Leg Shortened
- Adduction of Affected Leg
- External Rotation
- Deformity Along Lateral Side of the Hip if Fracture is Displaced
- Ecchymosis

NURSING CARE

- ✓ Dr's Orders
- Maintain Abduction
- Change Position q̄ 2 Hrs
- Avoid Affected Side
- Use Abduction Pillow Between Legs
- Out of Bed 1st Post-Op Day
- Cough & Deep Breath
- Monitor I & O
- Exercise When OK
- Client Teaching
- Avoid Extreme Hip Flexion
- Self Care Promotion
- Prevent External Rotation

POST OP CARE

Extremity For:
- Color
- Temperature
- Capillary Refill
- Distal Pulses
- Edema
- Sensation
- Motor Function
- Pain, Muscle Spasm

Prevent Neurovascular Impairment

Prevent adduction & external rotation of affected leg.

CLINICAL MANAGEMENT

- Treat coexisting medical disorders
  - Cardiac problems
  - Peripheral Vascular Disease
  - Neurologic disorders

TREATMENT

Depends on client condition & time since fracture was sustained. Also type of fracture

Surgery
(Internal fixation
  Pins - Screws - Plates
  Prosthetics)

Buck's Traction
to Relieve Spasms up to 24-48 Hours

ADDUCTION

EXTERNAL ROTATION

SHORTENING

NURSING CARE FOR SPRAINS AND STRAINS

R Rest

I Ice

C Compression

E Elevation

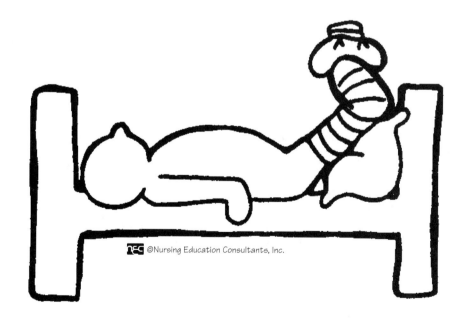

©Nursing Education Consultants, Inc.

Musculoskeletal
NursingEd.com

CARE OF PATIENT IN TRACTION

T — Temperature < Extremity / Infection

R — Ropes Hang Freely

A — Alignment

C — Circulation Check (5 P's)

T — Type & Location of Fracture

I — Increase Fluid Intake

O — Overhead Trapeze

N — No Weights On Bed Or Floor

©Nursing Education Consultants, Inc.

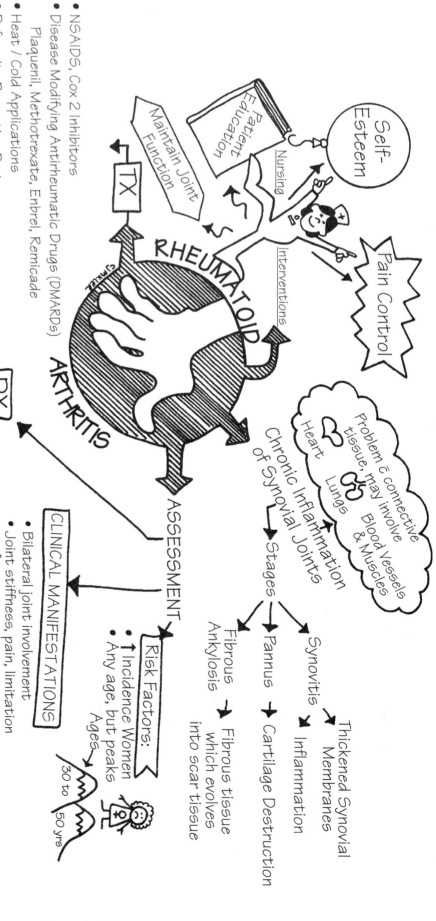

RHEUMATOID ARTHRITIS

Self-Esteem

Nursing
- Patient Education
- Maintain Joint Function
- Interventions
- Pain Control

TX
- NSAIDS, Cox 2 Inhibitors
- Disease Modifying Antirheumatic Drugs (DMARDs)
  - Plaquenil, Methotrexate, Enbrel, Remicade
- Heat / Cold Applications
- Deformity Preventing Devices
- Physical Therapy

COMPLICATIONS
Musculoskeletal - Hand Deformities, Flexion Contractures
Cardiac - Pericarditis - Myocarditis, Valve Involvement
Pulmonary - Fibrosis - Pneumonitis, Pleural Disease
Cataracts, Loss of Vision
Rheumatoid Nodules

DX
- ⊕ Serum Rheumatoid Factor
- ↑ ESR
- ↑ C-Reactive Protein
- Positive Antinuclear Antibody

Chronic Inflammation of Synovial Joints
- Problem c̄ connective tissue, may involve Heart, Lungs, Blood Vessels & Muscles

Stages
- Synovitis → Thickened Synovial Membranes → Inflammation
- Pannus → Cartilage Destruction
- Fibrous Ankylosis → Fibrous tissue which evolves into scar tissue

ASSESSMENT

Risk Factors:
- ↑ Incidence Women
- Any age, but peaks Ages 30 to 50 yrs

CLINICAL MANIFESTATIONS
- Bilateral joint involvement
- Joint stiffness, pain, limitation of movement
- Morning stiffness lasting >1hr
- Pain increases with movement
- Commonly affects joints of hands and fingers
- Extraarticular symptoms
  - ■ Rheumatoid nodules (located on extensor surface of joints)
  - ■ Sjögren's syndrome (decreased tearing, dry mouth, photosensitivity)
  - ■ Felty syndrome (splenomegaly, blood dyscrasias)

CARE OF

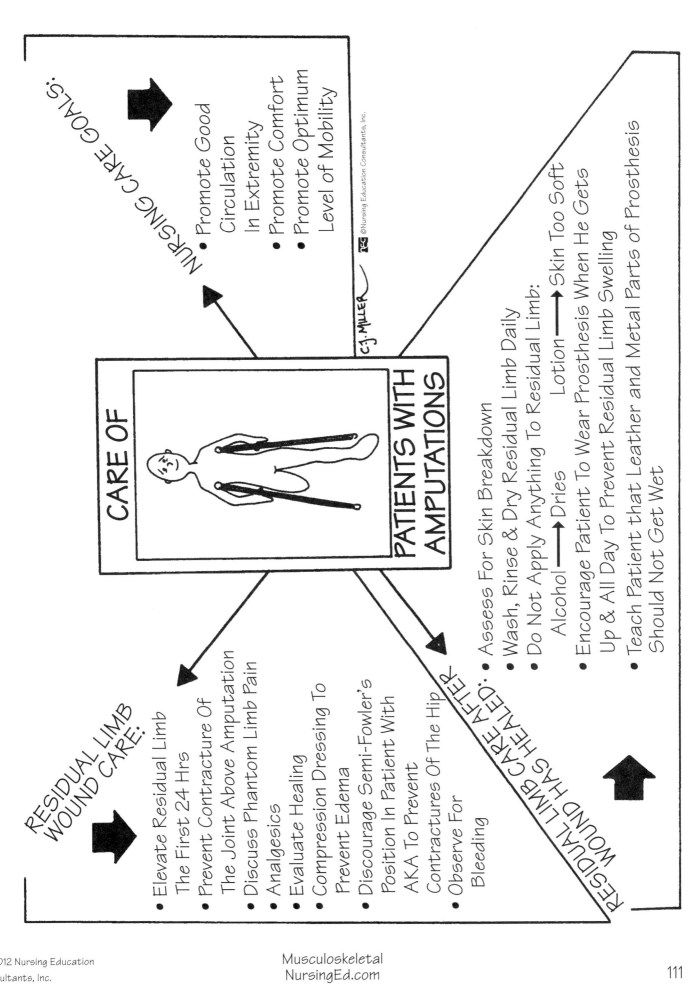

PATIENTS WITH AMPUTATIONS

NURSING CARE GOALS:

- Promote Good Circulation In Extremity
- Promote Comfort
- Promote Optimum Level of Mobility

RESIDUAL LIMB WOUND CARE:

- Elevate Residual Limb The First 24 Hrs
- Prevent Contracture Of The Joint Above Amputation
- Discuss Phantom Limb Pain
- Analgesics
- Evaluate Healing
- Compression Dressing To Prevent Edema
- Discourage Semi-Fowler's Position In Patient With AKA To Prevent Contractures Of The Hip
- Observe For Bleeding

RESIDUAL LIMB WOUND CARE AFTER:

- Assess For Skin Breakdown
- Wash, Rinse & Dry Residual Limb Daily
- Do Not Apply Anything To Residual Limb:
    - Alcohol → Dries   Lotion → Skin Too Soft
- Encourage Patient To Wear Prosthesis When He Gets Up & All Day To Prevent Residual Limb Swelling
- Teach Patient that Leather and Metal Parts of Prosthesis Should Not Get Wet

C.J. MILLER

©Nursing Education Consultants, Inc.

JOINT REPLACEMENTS

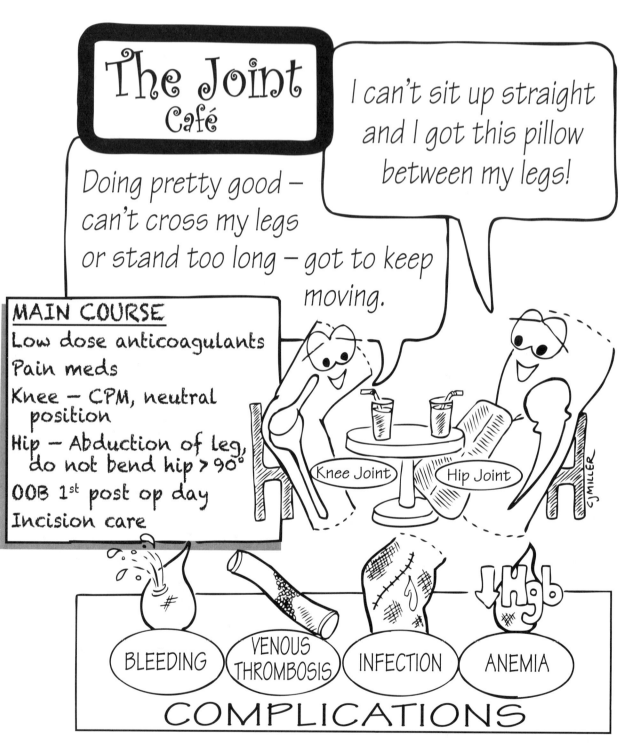

POST MASTECTOMY
NURSING CARE

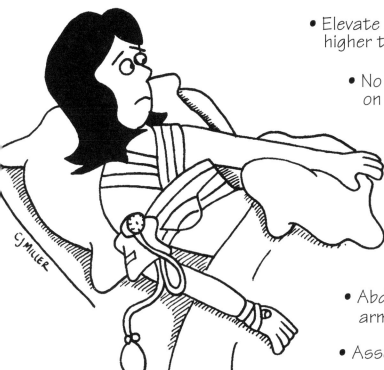

©Nursing Education Consultants, Inc.

- Elevate affected side with distal joint higher than proximal joint.

- No BP, injections or venipunctures on affected side.

- Watch for S & S of edema on affected arm. (edema may occur post op or years later)

- Lymphedema can occur any time after axillary node disection.

- Flexion and extension exercises of the hand in recovery.

- Abduction and external rotation arm exercises after wound has healed.

- Assess dressing for drainage.

- Assess wound drain for amount and color.

- Provide privacy when patient looks at incision.

- Chemotherapy, Radiation therapy.

- Monitor for Complications – hemorrhage, hematoma, lymphedema, infection, postmastectomy pain syndrome.

- Psychological concerns:
    Altered body image
    Altered sexuality
    Fear of disease outcome

TURP
(Transurethral Resection of the Prostate)

- Continuous or Intermittent Bladder Irrigation (C.B.I.) (Usually DC'd after 24 hours, if No Clots).   Murphy Drip

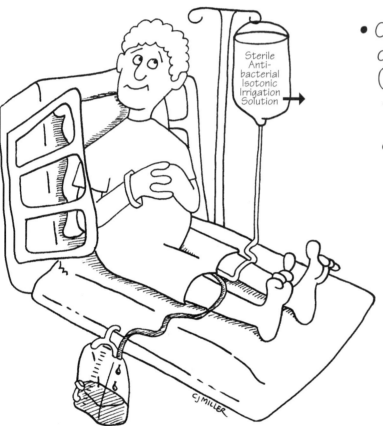

Sterile Anti-bacterial Isotonic Irrigation Solution →

©Nursing Education Consultants, Inc.

- Close observation of drainage system- (↑Bladder Distention causes Pain & Bleeding).

- Maintain Catheter Patency

- Bladder Spasms

- Pain Control: Analgesics & ↓ Activity first 24 hours.

- Avoid straining with BMs ↑ Fiber diet & Laxatives.

- Complications:
  - Hemorrhage - Bleeding should gradually to light pink in 24 hrs.
  - Urinary Incontinence - Kegel Exercises
  - Infections - ↑Fluids
  - Prevent Deep Vein Thrombosis
  - Sequential compression stockings
  - Discourage sitting for prolonged periods

URINARY TRACT INFECTION (UTI)

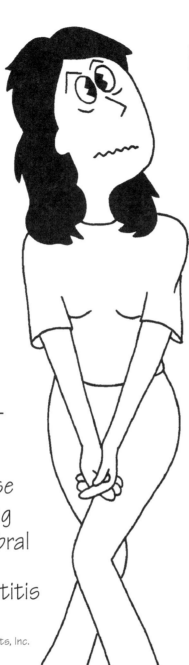

CYSTITIS:

- Frequency
- Urgency
- Suprapubic Pain
- Dysuria
- Hematuria
- Fever
- Confusion
  - in Older Adults

PYELONEPHRITIS:

- Flank Pain
- Dysuria
- Mild Fatigue, Malaise
- Chills, Fever, Vomiting
- Pain At Costovertebral Angle
- Same S & S as Cystitis

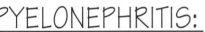

©Nursing Education Consultants, Inc.

DX: →
Dipstick for
Leukocyte Esterase
and Nitrates
Midstream UA / C&S
↑Risk in older adults

TX: →
Antibiotics
↑ Fluid Intake
Prevention

NURSING GOALS:

Cystitis

- Symptomatic Relief
- Teaching & Prevention
- Showers Better Than Baths
- Perineal Cleansing "Front To Back"
- Voiding After Intercourse
- Anti-Microbial Therapy
- No Scented Toilet Paper
- No Perfumes, Etc. to Perineal Area
- Empty Bladder Regularly

Pyelonephritis

- May Require Hospitalization
- Severe Cases – IV Antibiotics Initially
- Monitor for Urosepsis to Prevent Septic Shock

RENAL CALCULI

- ↑ Incidence in Males

- Nausea & Vomiting

- Agonizing Flank Pain
  May Radiate To:
   Groin
   Testicles
   Abdominal Area

- Sharp, Sudden,
  Severe Pain:
  (May be intermittent
  depending on
  stone movement)

- Hematuria

- Dysuria

- Urinary Frequency

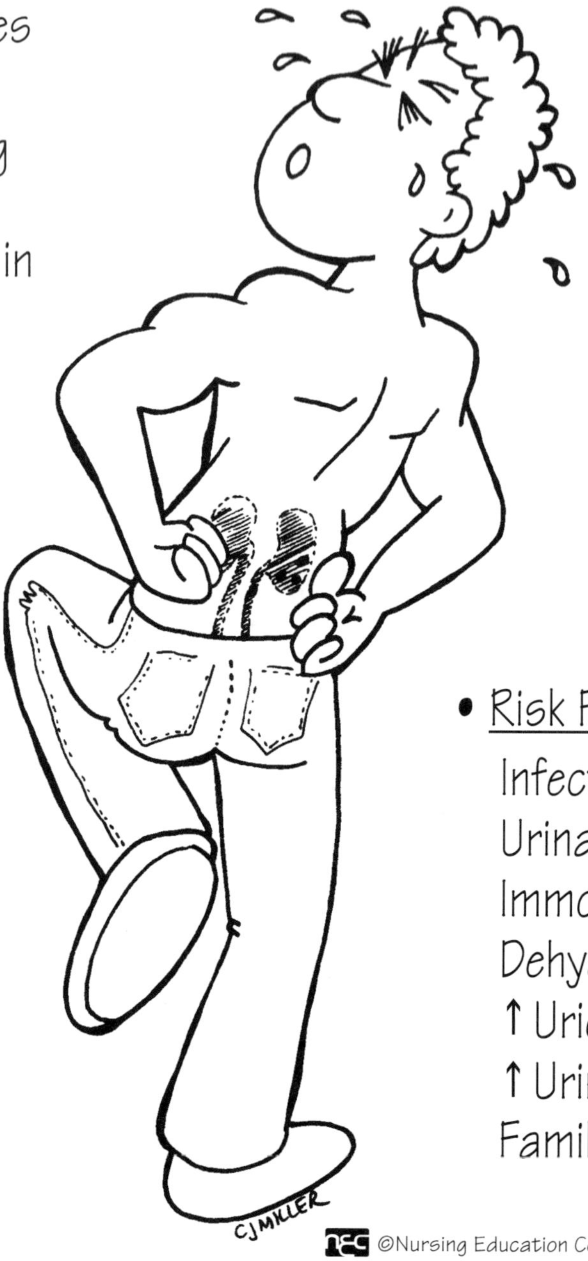

- Diagnosis
  Ultrasound, CT Scar
  IVP
  Renal Stone Analysi
  Retrograde pyelogra
  Cystsocopy
  Measure Urine pH

- Risk Factors - Etiology
   Infection
   Urinary Stasis & Retention
   Immobility
   Dehydration
   ↑ Uric Acid
   ↑ Urinary Oxalate
   Family History

CJMILLER

ACUTE KIDNEY INJURY (AKI)

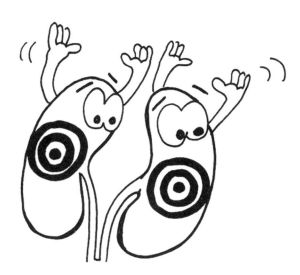

R isk – First Stage of AKI – Creatinine ↑ x 1.5 or GFR ↓ 25%

I njury – Second Stage – Creatinine ↑ x 2 or GFR ↓ 50%

F ailure – Third Stage – Creatinine ↑ x 3
   or GFR ↓ 75% or Creatinine > 4mg/dL

L oss – Fourth Stage – Persistent Acute
   Kidney Failure; Loss of Function > 4 wk

E nd-Stage Kidney Disease – Complete Loss
   of Kidney Function > 3 mo

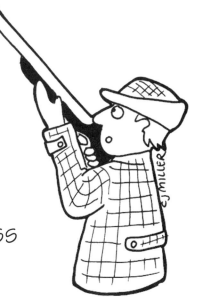

ACUTE KIDNEY INJURY (AKI)
- SIGNS & SYMPTOMS -

Oliguric Phase

- Oliguria - <400mL/day; occurs within 1-7 days of kidney injury
- Urinalysis — casts, RBCs, WBCs, sp gr fixated at 1.010
- Metabolic Acidosis
- Hyperkalemia and Hyponatremia
- Elevated BUN and Creatinine
- Fatigue & Malaise

Diuretic Phase

- Gradual ↑ in urine output - 1-3 L/day; may reach 3-5 L/day
- Hypovolemia, Dehydration
- Hypotension
- BUN and Creatinine Levels Begin to Normalize

Recovery Phase

- Begins when GFR Increases
- BUN and Creatinine Levels Plateau, then ↓

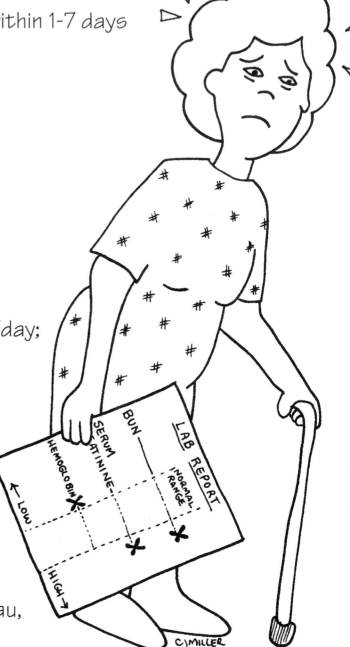

CJMILLER

CHRONIC KIDNEY DISEASE (CKD)

ESRD – END-STAGE KIDNEY [RENAL] DISEASE
↓ 15 ml/min GFR

Neurologic
Weakness / Fatigue
Headache
Sleep Disturbances

Cardiovascular
↑BP
Pitting Edema
Periorbital Edema
Heart Faulure
Pericarditis
Peripheral Artery
  Disease

• Pulmonary
  Pulmonary Edema
  Uremic Pleuritis
  Pneumonia

• GI
  Ammonia Odor to Breath
  Metallic Taste
  Mouth / Gum Ulcerations
  Anorexia
  Nausea / Vomiting
  GI Bleeding

• Psychologic
  Withdrawn
  Behavior Changes
  Depression

  • Hematologic
    Anemia
    Bleeding Tendencies
    Infection

• Fld/Lytes - ↑ Potassium
  Acid/Base - Metabolic
              Acidosis

• Skin
  Dry Flaky
  Pruritus
  Ecchymosis
  Yellow-gray
    skin color

• Musculoskeletal
  Cramps
  Renal
    Osteodystrophy
  Bone Pain

CJMILLER

Hemodialysis

• Evaluate access site for patency & signs of infection.
• **DO NOT** take BP, insert IV line, or perform venipuncture in extremity with vascular access.

©Nursing Education Consultants, Inc.

PHYSIOLOGIC CHANGES IN PREGNANCY

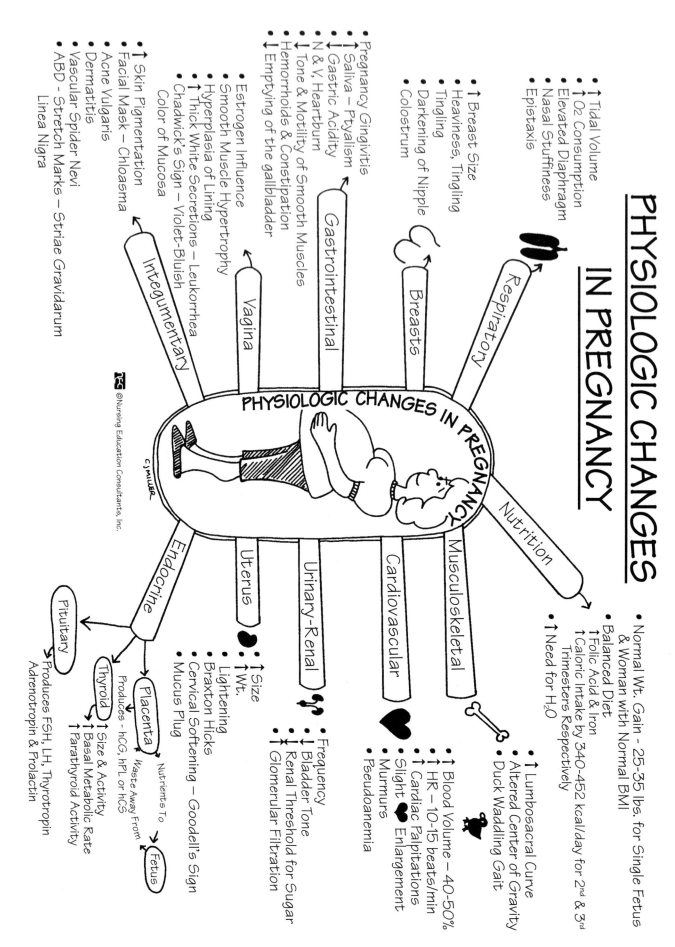

PHYSIOLOGIC CHANGES IN PREGNANCY

C J MILLER

© Nursing Education Consultants, Inc.

Respiratory
- ↑ Tidal Volume
- ↑ O₂ Consumption
- Elevated Diaphragm
- Nasal Stuffiness
- Epistaxis

Breasts
- ↑ Breast Size
- Heaviness, Tingling
- Tingling
- Darkening of Nipple
- Colostrum

Gastrointestinal
- Pregnancy Gingivitis
- ↑ Saliva – Ptyalism
- ↓ Gastric Acidity
- N & V, Heartburn
- ↓ Tone & Motility of Smooth Muscles
- Hemorrhoids & Constipation
- ↓ Emptying of the gallbladder

Vagina
- Estrogen Influence
- Smooth Muscle Hypertrophy
- Hyperplasia of Lining
- ↑ Thick White Secretions – Leukorrhea
- Chadwick's Sign – Violet-Bluish Color of Mucosa

Integumentary
- ↑ Skin Pigmentation
- Facial Mask – Chloasma
- Acne Vulgaris
- Dermatitis
- Vascular Spider Nevi
- ABD - Stretch Marks – Striae Gravidarum
- Linea Nigra

Nutrition
- Normal Wt. Gain - 25-35 lbs. for Single Fetus & Woman with Normal BMI
- Balanced Diet
- ↑ Folic Acid & Iron
- ↑ Caloric Intake by 340-452 kcal/day for 2ⁿᵈ & 3ʳᵈ Trimesters Respectively
- ↑ Need for H₂O

Musculoskeletal
- ↑ Lumbosacral Curve
- Altered Center of Gravity
- Duck Waddling Gait
- Pseudoanemia

Cardiovascular
- ↑ Blood Volume – 40-50%
- ↑ HR – 10-15 beats/min
- ↑ Cardiac Palpitations
- Slight ♥ Enlargement
- Murmurs
- Pseudoanemia

Urinary-Renal
- ↑ Frequency
- ↓ Bladder Tone
- ↓ Renal Threshold for Sugar
- ↑ Glomerular Filtration

Uterus
- ↑ Size
- ↑ Wt.
- Lightening
- Braxton Hicks
- Cervical Softening – Goodell's Sign
- Mucus Plug

Endocrine

Pituitary
- Produces FSH, LH, Thyrotropin Adrenotropin & Prolactin

Thyroid
- ↑ Size & Activity
- ↑ Basal Metabolic Rate
- ↑ Parathyroid Activity

Placenta
- Produces – hCG, hPL or hCS

Waste Away From
Nutrients To
→ Fetus

© Nursing Education Consultants, Inc.

PRENATAL CARE

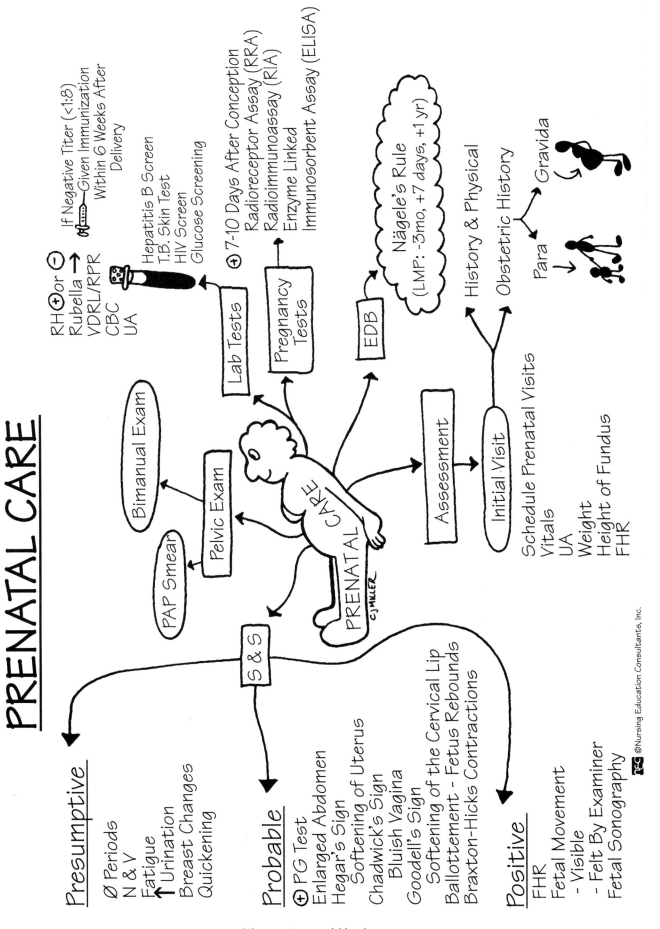

Presumptive
Ø Periods
N & V
Fatigue
↑ Urination
Breast Changes
Quickening

Probable
⊕ PG Test
Enlarged Abdomen
Hegar's Sign
Softening of Uterus
Chadwick's Sign
Bluish Vagina
Goodell's Sign
Softening of the Cervical Lip
Ballottement - Fetus Rebounds
Braxton-Hicks Contractions

Positive
FHR
Fetal Movement
- Visible
- Felt By Examiner
Fetal Sonography

S & S

PAP Smear

Pelvic Exam

Bimanual Exam

Lab Tests

RH ⊕ or ⊖
Rubella
VDRL/RPR
CBC
UA

If Negative Titer (<1:8)
Given Immunization
Within 6 Weeks After
Delivery

Hepatitis B Screen
T.B. Skin Test
HIV Screen
Glucose Screening

Pregnancy Tests

⊕ 7-10 Days After Conception
Radioreceptor Assay (RRA)
Radioimmunoassay (RIA)
Enzyme Linked
Immunosorbent Assay (ELISA)

EDB

Nägele's Rule
(LMP: -3mo, +7 days, +1 yr)

Assessment

History & Physical
Obstetric History

Gravida

Para

Initial Visit

Schedule Prenatal Visits
Vitals
UA
Weight
Height of Fundus
FHR

CJ MILLER

PRENATAL CARE

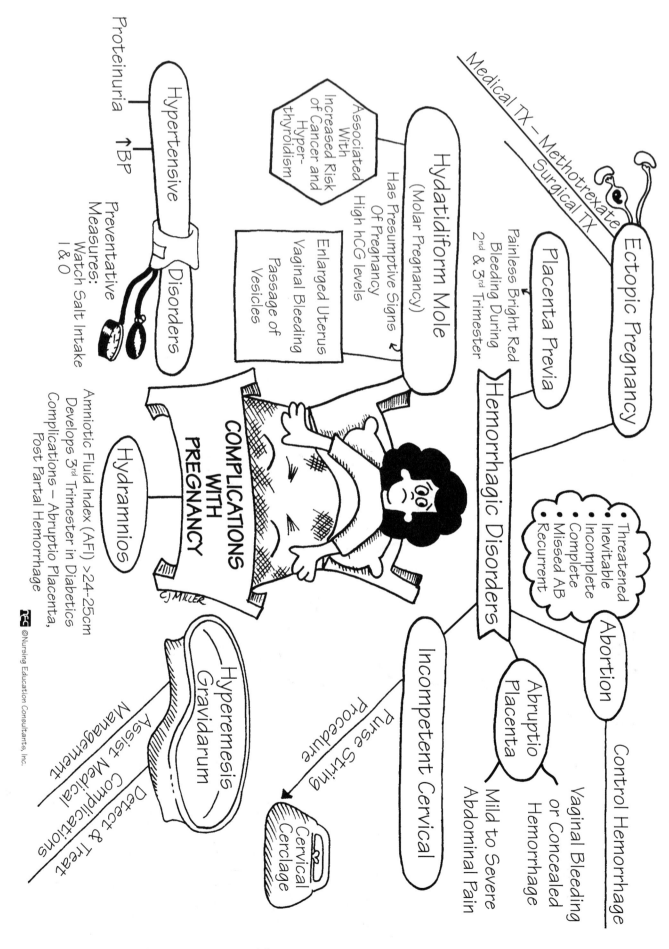

COMPLICATIONS WITH PREGNANCY

Hypertensive Disorders
- Proteinuria
- ↑BP
- Preventative Measures: Watch Salt Intake I & O

Hydatidiform Mole (Molar Pregnancy)
- Associated With Increased Risk of Cancer and Hyper-thyroidism
- Has Presumptive Signs Of Pregnancy
- High hCG levels
- Enlarged Uterus
- Vaginal Bleeding
- Passage of Vesicles

Placenta Previa
- Painless Bright Red Bleeding During 2nd & 3rd Trimester

Ectopic Pregnancy
- Medical TX – Methotrexate
- Surgical TX

Hemorrhagic Disorders

Abortion
- Threatened
- Inevitable
- Incomplete
- Complete
- Missed AB
- Recurrent
- Control Hemorrhage

Abruptio Placenta
- Mild to Severe Abdominal Pain
- Vaginal Bleeding or Concealed Hemorrhage

Incompetent Cervical
- Purse String Procedure
- Cervical Cerclage

Hyperemesis Gravidarum
- Detect & Treat
- Assist Medical Management Complications

Hydramnios
- Amniotic Fluid Index (AFI) >24-25cm
- Develops 3rd Trimester in Diabetics
- Complications – Abruptio Placenta, Post Partal Hemorrhage

CJ MILLER

NON-STRESS TEST

3 Negatives in a row to interpret results
of non-stress test

N Non-Reactive

N Non-Stress is

N Not Good

ASSESSMENT TESTS FOR FETAL WELL-BEING

BIOPHYSICAL PROFILE *

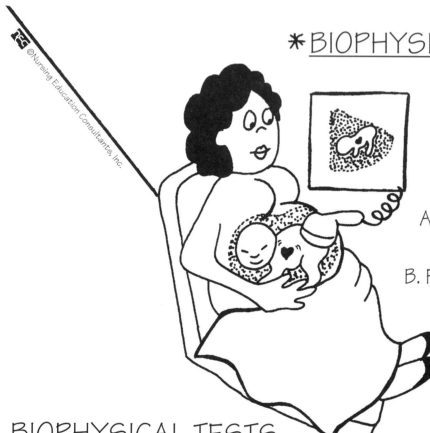

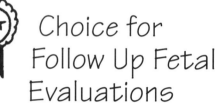 Choice for Follow Up Fetal Evaluations

A. Fetal Breathing Movements - 1 episode of 30 sec. in 30 min

B. Fetal Tone - At least 1 episode of extremity extension & flexion

C. Body Movement - 3 episodes over 30 min.

D. Amniotic Fluid Volume - At least 1 pocket measure 2cm in 2 perpendicular plan

E. Non-Stress Test - Reactive - FHR ↑ with activity.

Each has a possible score of 2

Max Score = 10 ☺

BIOPHYSICAL TESTS

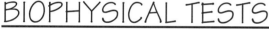

- Daily Fetal Movement Count (DFMC)
- Ultrasonography
- Biophysical Profile (BPP)*
- MRI

BIOCHEMICAL TESTS

- Amniocentesis
- Chorionic Villus Sampling (CVS)
- Percutaneous Umbilical Blood Sampling (PUBS)
- Maternal Serum Alpha-Fetoprotein (MSAFP)
- Indirect Coombs Test

Maternity and Newborn
NursingEd.com

HELLP SYNDROME
(Preeclampsia with Liver Involvement)

Hemolysis
Elevated **L**iver Function Tests
Low **P**latelet Count

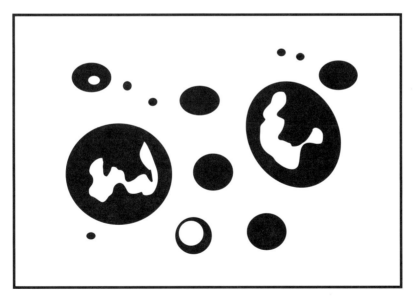

©Nursing Education Consultants, Inc.

STAGES OF LABOR

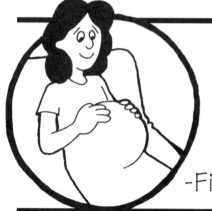

(Stage of Cervical Dilation) Begins with onset of regular contractions and ends with complete dilation.

Latent ➝ Active ➝ Transitional
(0-3 cm)   (4-7 cm)   (8-10 cm)

-First Stage -

(Stage of Expulsion) Begins with complete cervical dilation and ends with delivery of fetus.

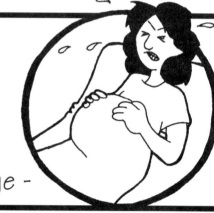

- Second Stage -

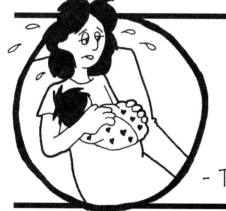

(Placental Stage) Begins immediately after fetus is born and ends when the placenta is delivered.

- Third Stage -

(Maternal Homeostatic Stabilization Stage) Begins after the delivery of the placenta and continues for one to four hours after delivery.

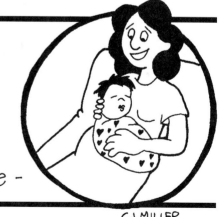

- Fourth Stage -

C.J. MILLER

Maternity and Newborn
NursingEd.com

POSTPARTUM ASSESSMENT

B **B**reasts

U **U**terus

B **B**owels

B **B**ladder

L **L**ochia

E **E**pisiotomy/Laceration/
C-Section Incision

EVALUATION OF EPISIOTOMY HEALING

R **R**edness

E **E**dema

E **E**cchymosis

D **D**ischarge, **D**rainage

A **A**pproximation

©Nursing Education Consultants, Inc.

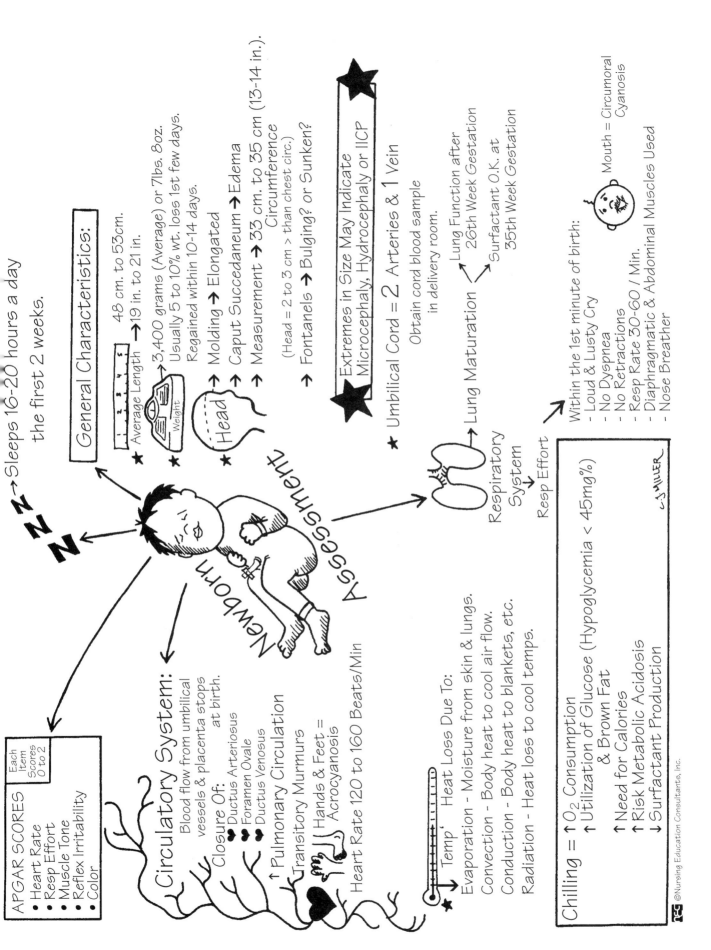

Newborn Assessment

Z Z Z → Sleeps 16-20 hours a day the first 2 weeks.

General Characteristics:

★ Average Length → 48 cm. to 53cm. → 19 in. to 21 in.

★ Weight → 3,400 grams (Average) or 7lbs. 8oz. Usually 5 to 10% wt. loss 1st few days. Regained within 10-14 days.

Head

★ Molding → Elongated
→ Caput Succedaneum → Edema
→ Measurement → 33 cm. to 35 cm (13-14 in.). Circumference
(Head = 2 to 3 cm > than chest circ.)
→ Fontanels → Bulging? or Sunken?

★ Extremes in Size May Indicate Microcephaly, Hydrocephaly or IICP

★ Umbilical Cord = 2 Arteries & 1 Vein
Obtain cord blood sample in delivery room.

Respiratory System

→ Lung Maturation → Lung Function after 26th Week Gestation
→ Surfactant O.K. at 35th Week Gestation

Resp Effort

Within the 1st minute of birth:
- Loud & Lusty Cry
- No Dyspnea
- No Retractions
- Resp Rate 30-60 / Min.
- Diaphragmatic & Abdominal Muscles Used
- Nose Breather

Mouth = Circumoral Cyanosis

APGAR SCORES
Each Item Scores 0 to 2
- Heart Rate
- Resp Effort
- Muscle Tone
- Reflex Irritability
- Color

Circulatory System:

Blood flow from umbilical vessels & placenta stops at birth.

Closure Of:
- Ductus Arteriosus
- Foramen Ovale
- Ductus Venosus

↑ Pulmonary Circulation
Transitory Murmurs
↓ Hands & Feet = Acrocyanosis

Heart Rate 120 to 160 Beats/Min

Temp↑ Heat Loss Due To:
Evaporation - Moisture from skin & lungs.
Convection - Body heat to cool air flow.
Conduction - Body heat to blankets, etc.
Radiation - Heat loss to cool temps.

Chilling = ↑O₂ Consumption
↑ Utilization of Glucose (Hypoglycemia < 45mg%) & Brown Fat
↑ Need for Calories
↑ Risk Metabolic Acidosis
↓ Surfactant Production

C.J. MILLER

- HIGH RISK NEWBORN -
NURSING INTERVENTIONS

TEMPERATURE

☆ Minimize Cold Stress.

☆ Maintain Skin Temp. 36.1° - 36.7°C (96.8° - 97.7°F)

☆ Continuously Monitor Temp.

☆ Prevent Rapid Warming or Cooling.

☆ Use A Cap To Prevent Heat Loss From Head.

FOOD & FLUIDS

☆ Monitor For Hypoglycemia.

☆ Assess Tolerance Of Oral Or Tube Feedings.

☆ Monitor Hydration Closely.

☆ Assess For Gastric Residual, Bowel Sounds,

☆ Change In Stool Pattern, Abdominal Girth.

☆ Monitor Weight Gain Or Loss.

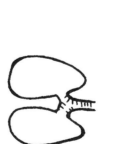

RESP FUNCTION

☆ Position ↑ O_2 - Semiprone/Side Lying.

☆ Maintain Resp Tract Patency.

☆ Stimulate → Remind to Breathe.

☆ Monitor O_2 Therapy.

☆ Assess Resp Effort.
- Grunting
- Nasal Flaring
- Cyanosis
- Apnea

TRACHEAL - ESOPHAGEAL FISTULA

(3C's)

C. Choking

C. Coughing

C. Cyanosis

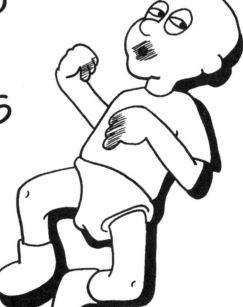

©Nursing Education Consultants, Inc.

Malformation of the Hip Due to Imperfect Development of the Femoral Head, Acetabulum, or Both. (Most often assessed at birth.)

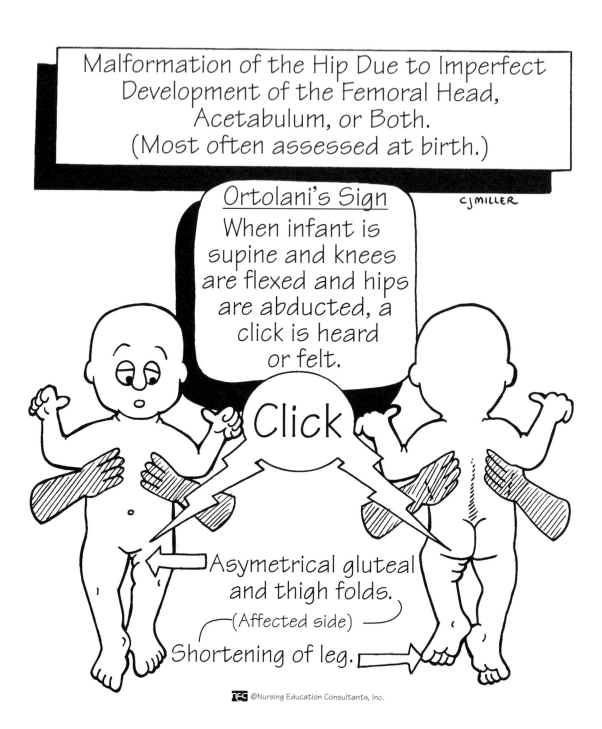

CJMILLER

Ortolani's Sign

When infant is supine and knees are flexed and hips are abducted, a click is heard or felt.

Click

Asymetrical gluteal and thigh folds. (Affected side)

Shortening of leg.

©Nursing Education Consultants, Inc.

CLEFT LIP - POST OP CARE

C Choking

L Lie on Back

E Evaluate Airway

F Feed Slowly

T Teaching

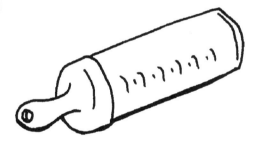

L Larger Nipple Opening

I Incidence ↑ Males

P Prevent Crust Formation
Prevent Aspiration

 ©Nursing Education Consultants, Inc.

IMMINENT DEADLINE STRESS DISORDER
(I.D.S.D.)

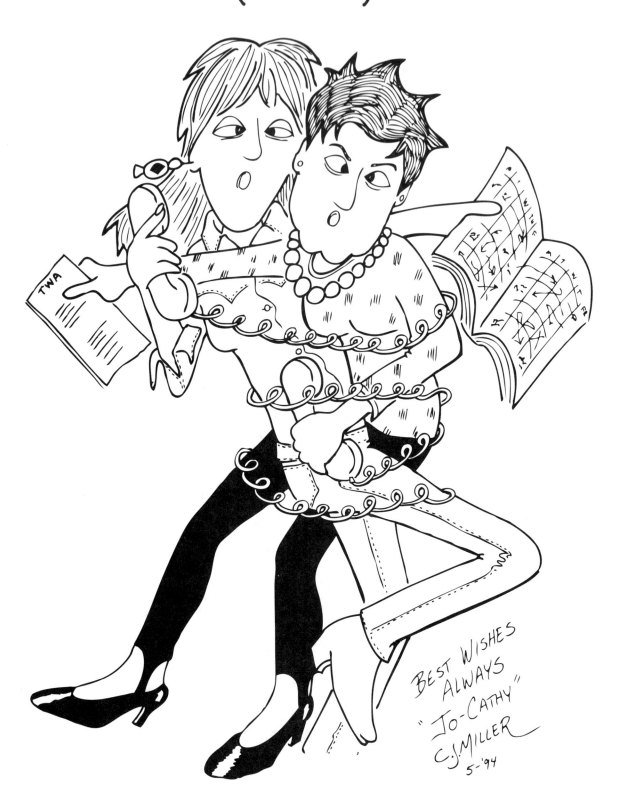

134

Memory Notebook of Nursing, Vol. 1 - 5th ed.
NursingEd.com

© 2012 Nursing Educat
Consultants, I

INDEX

2012 Nursing Education
sultants, Inc.

Memory Notebook of Nursing, Vol. 1 - 5th ed.
NursingEd.com

135

2012 Nursing Education
sultants, Inc.

Memory Notebook of Nursing, Vol. 1 - 5th ed.
NursingEd.com

137

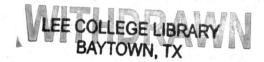
Memory Notebook of Nursing, Vol. 1 - 5th ed.
NursingEd.com

© 2012 Nursing Educat
Consultants,